HERBAL MEDICINE

SIMPLE AND EFFECTIVE NATURAL
REMEDIES TO HEAL COMMON AILMENTS

BY JOSEPH BOSNER

© Copyright 2019 - All rights reserved.

The content contained within this book may not be reproduced, duplicated or transmitted without direct written permission from the author or the publisher.

Under no circumstances will any blame or legal responsibility be held against the publisher, or author, for any damages, reparation, or monetary loss due to the information contained within this book. Either directly or indirectly.

Legal Notice:

This book is copyright protected. This book is only for personal use. You cannot amend, distribute, sell, use, quote or paraphrase any part, or the content within this book, without the consent of the author or publisher.

Disclaimer Notice:

Please note the information contained within this document is for educational and entertainment purposes only. All effort has been executed to present accurate, up to date, and reliable, complete information. No warranties of any kind are declared or implied. Readers acknowledge that the author is not engaging in the rendering of legal, financial, medical or professional advice. The content within this book has been derived from various sources.

HERBAL MEDICINE

Please consult a licensed professional before attempting any techniques outlined in this book.

By reading this document, the reader agrees that under no circumstances is the author responsible for any losses, direct or indirect, which are incurred as a result of the use of information contained within this document, including, but not limited to, — errors, omissions, or inaccuracies.

HERBAL MEDICINE

Table of Contents

Introduction V

Chapter 1 Herbal Medicine History... 1

Chapter 2 How To Use Medicinal Herbs..................................... 16

    BASIC BROTH RECIPE 25
    BASIC SOUP RECIPE 26
    BASIC STEW RECIPE.. 27
    BASIC SALVE RECIPE 29
    BASIC ESSENCES RECIPE... 30
    BASIC EXTRACTION RECIPE.. 32

Chapter 3 Selecting The Best Herbs.. 37

Chapter 4 Essential Herbs.. 43

Chapter 5 Remedies And Recipes.. 93

    BASIC COUGH SYRUP RECIPE 96
    BASIC THROAT COAT RECIPE (FOR SORE THROATS) 97
    BASIC COLD AND FLU REMEDY... 98
    WARM AND COZY REMEDY... 99
    ASTRINGENT RECIPE... 100
    BASIC SALVE FOR CUTS, BURNS AND BRUISES 101
    TONIC FOR BOWEL DISCOMFORT 102
    TONIC FOR VITALITY.. 103

Chapter 6 Applications 105

Conclusion 113

INTRODUCTION

The world was always aware of herbal remedies, even in this current day and age. As old as human beings are as a species, we have known the world of plant medicine. Herbal remedies always asked for a way to become one with our journey through life as we learned through the process of trial and error over the course of thousands and thousands of years, which herb worked well for what ailment, and also which were going to set you up in an early coffin.

As far back as the Neanderthals, we had known the use of certain tools and powerful drugs, even including alcohol when it was the product of rotten and fermented fruits from trees. No one knew what they were walking into back in those days, when they ate a poisonous plant; it only seemed like a piece of food they could use to sustain life.

When we all began to evolve into the world of agriculture and were able to ask more questions through language and writing, we were able to find a frame of reference and create an herbal dictionary to help us all understand the Universal qualities of each plant, root, leaf, or flower remedy.

Many herbalists today don't use the ancient, old-wife's tales and wisdom from the days of yore because of how the Age of Reason told a new tale of science and mathematics, letting medicinal folklore get the boot in favor of a more studied approach to all life and all manner of living well and healthfully.

In today's market, most herbal remedies are replaced by over the counter, prescription drugs and all they have assisted with is the creation of even more traumatic and deathly illnesses because of how enormously against or natural bodies they actually are.

We are not made for those kinds of drugs, and all of our herbal medicine worked before we started to judge and criticize the knowledge of the Great Mother herself, Earth. All of her herbal offspring are how we will actually heal ourselves well and return to our original bodies in a healthy way. Few people alive today have the actual remedies for how our Universal energies would like to be handled as we no longer listen to the magic of the plant world.

Only certain individuals, these days, and small groups of people who worship the assistance of Mother Nature's medicine cabinet, know who each little plant is and what they will offer you as a remedy. Here in these pages, you will find a true account of all of the knowledge you need to get you started with learning the basics of natural herbal remedies and how to use them. You will enjoy a history of how we have lived side by side with these medicines throughout our evolution and how we came to disregard them in favor of pharmaceuticals.

The protection of this knowledge and this wisdom is in your capable hands and as you look through these pages, enjoy knowing that you are tapping into the ancient wisdom of the world and of the Earth Mother herself.

HERBAL MEDICINE

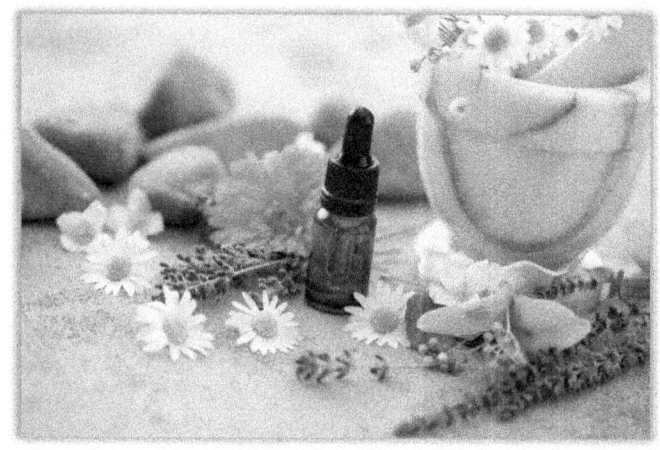

CHAPTER 1

HERBAL MEDICINE HISTORY

Ancient wisdom was always about a medicine cabinet and how to use it; the theories of how to keep well and stay alive have lived alongside human beings throughout many cultures and ages in history. Only a few lifetimes ago, a select group of people held a high and mighty dollar amount over the head of a certain and very valuable herbal remedy that lost its favor with all of the popular diets and journals of medicine published in the modern era leading to a miseducation by a variety of doctors and medical professionals: salt.

You may not think at first that this element is an herbal remedy; however, it has always been treated as one throughout the ages and only lost its favor in the medical world when doctors began to treat people with the use of prescription medications and over the counter pharmaceuticals. This ancient remedy has always been of great value to the health of the human body, but only when the body is not congested with other materials that hinder its ability to heal.

HERBAL MEDICINE

Diet and exercise are the current trend with how to stay in good shape and have a healthy life, however what many of these current trends question without any actual affirmation or affective knowledge is how to ask for an energetic balance in their bodies with the right connection of herbal remedies with your current health plans.

Many people have discovered alternative medicines to work with a variety of diseases and difficulties in the whole body without reflecting on the fact that none of these ailments and diseases actually existed over 1000 years ago. As our civilization announced the progress of creating highly processed foods and sugars into the lives of all people in civilized cultures, the whole world began to see the advent of curious and unknown diseases that were not around as much in the cultures of the past. The influx of new disease began simply with the agriculture and food demand of two things: the grain mill and the whole cup of sugar.

Since the beginning of "daily bread" and a spoonful of sugar asking the medicine to go down, we have culturally and globally found a direct link to how ailments, food, substances, and chemicals all play a major part in the whole health of the human body. Not many people truly understand how toxic and abusive daily quantities of wheat products and sugary treats can be to the integrity of the whole system and even when you treat all of the diseases and ailments of the body with prescribed medications from your family physician, you will cure nothing without identifying this major cause of whole wellness disturbance and internal malfunction.

Some sugars and wheat-related products can be beneficial to a regular diet when utilized in smaller quantities. Similar to the wheat grain in its ability to puff up and add texture and girth to the belly, corn has had a major use in historical diets and it wasn't until the very recent past that corn farmers began to destroy the integrity of the health benefits of corn by working at half its capacity in growth and value to produce larger quantities of it to feed more cows to make more beef to feed more people.

Corn had a highly nutritious quality before we all tampered with its quality and health benefits and currently, only some heirloom varieties still contain the best nutrition for human consumption. Unfortunately, most store-bought products that contain corn, which is a lot, are not of this variety and the only place you will find this heirloom herbal corn remedy is at your local farmer's market or grown in your own backyard.

Sugar, on the other hand, is only healing or valuable to the human body in its purest form: fruit and honey, and that's it. No other version of sugar will ever be healthy for the human body unless you are putting it into an herbal sugar body scrub to help your skin find a cleansing exfoliation, and it is not likely that our culture and societies all over the world will let go of their addiction to sweet things created with this harmful product.

HERBAL MEDICINE

Your body is stripped of its vitality when you implement sugar into your daily diet and when you remove sugar from how you eat, your body has lost a lot of its vitality and essential nutrient density. The best way to replenish this loss is through a very commonly known herbal concoction that has been around for ages and ages: bone broth.

It may not seem like an herbal remedy as it is made, not from plants, flowers or roots, but from bones, simmered for hours with other plant-based herbs, like carrots, onions, celery, bay leaf, thyme and rosemary, to collect all of the vital energies required to relieve your body of its severe loss of nutrients from a sugary diet.

The history of herbal medicine dates back to the time of agriculture. After the hunter-gatherer societies pinned themselves down to a location and began to learn from the Earth how to grow what they needed in one place, they began to form a closer connection to which plants fed what need in the body, how much of it to use, what could poison you, kill you or make you ill, and how to prepare each one in the most beneficial manner.

Some of these remedies and concoctions still exist in today's modern world, and bone broth, traditionally used as a medicine, is now only a base for soups and is mostly a processed food item with unnatural ingredients that comes in a can or a box. The real medicine comes from the living, herbal remedies, plucked from the garden and tossed into the boiling water alongside the bones to create the perfect potion for healing a loss of energy and nutrients, and health in the sick, infirm, weak and unwell.

The best herbal remedies have been known to heal a lot of issues and have been utilized by old world physicians and witch doctors from the days of yore when people still bought their groceries from their own home gardens and from their own livestock of animals. Plenty of people had sickness in those days because there wasn't a lot of understanding about how to clean the self or their tools that they used to cook, wash, bath, and heal themselves. Most of the time, people just used a small amount of salt and some rubbing powders in order to scrub their dirty dishes and clean their underarms, fingers, and toes and back then, a bath a month was more likely than a hot shower every day.

Soap didn't find its regular place in society until the 18th century, and even then, only the wealthy lords and ladies were able to afford its beautiful essences and perfumes. All of the poor people had to use a strictly small amount of soap that was so caustic that it could burn your flesh if you put too much on and it wasn't until a short while later that lye soap was mixed efficiently with lards, and fats to help it work more effectively and less harshly on the skin.

When we all began to use soap, the need for herbal remedies all of the time lessened and became a greater portion of an old way of doing things with regard to health and the body, because as soap became popularized, so too did scientific medicines and an advance in the tools and technology to question and dissect ailments, diseases and injuries of the tissues, bones and ligaments.

Dissecting a patient after death was a new way for "medicine men" to determine a cause of disease and eventual death in a person; it led to a new way of looking at health and the physical body. Herbal remedies were altered to involve a much more fashionable as well as fantastical reality as more and more people allowed for these "medical professionals" to practice their theories and hypotheses on the human body and its ailments.

In order to please the royalty of the day, the scientists who worked in medicine, who became known as 'doctors,' created a suitable amount of theoretical remedies to suit the fashion of the day which was always about impressing the King and/or Queen and their court. It wasn't actually based in well-researched or well-documented cases of healing; it was more often a fad to ask for the favor of the royal family as it was the most important gift of all time to be in the favor of the king or queen's court.

All of these 'fad remedies' were based on the knowledge from the not too distant past when we were all acquainted through our closeness with the world of herbs, plants, flowers, trees, and animals to the power of natural medicine. The benefit of this knowledge was always kept close to several people who lived on the outskirts and worked the land for food and money and behaved in a manner of allowing the herbs to tell you how to heal instead of the other way around, with the "doctors" telling you how to heal your body's ailments.

Only the herbs know the actual way to heal the human body and most doctors, as they are still called today, only work with their own intellectual beliefs about health and well-being, instead of allowing the power and magic of herbs to coach them into the best way to help someone's ailments and health concerns.

All of the herbs that you have heard of in the common garden are a medicinal remedy and each has a unique way of healing that is different from all of the rest. There are plenty of common herbs and also a lot that you may not even recognize as being called an herbal medicine. Take for example the plantain; it bears a banana like fruit and also has thick and powerful leaves that have a lot of benefit to your colon and all of the digestive diseases of that area. All of the plant would be beneficial to the digestive tract, but it is the leaves that have the most beneficial impact on this area of the body and have the most common benefit to the colon than most other remedies around the doctor's office.

Each plantain leaf has a potent mineral and acidic content that, when brewed as a tea from the dried leaves and consumed at regular intervals during digestive problems, will cause a passage of toxins out of the body that are collecting in the colon and causing a severe disturbance in the energy of the bowels. Each sip of tea travels through the body and displaces the back up of wastes that the body has trapped within the end of the digestive system.

Overall, a tea remedy has been the ancient symbol of medicine that has still found a powerful footing in all cultures across the centuries and as of today remains the most heavily consumed beverage, after alcohol. The healing power of a tea concoction still benefits all of us. Most people these days use it as a caffeinated alternative to coffee, however, many tea shops have a variety of herbal teas that support a lot of internal body issues and promote an internal balance that can only be achieved through the use of certain herbs on a regular, daily basis.

Brand name beverages, like Coca-Cola and Pepsi, were once a blend of strong herbs with a lot of healing benefit but were over-manipulated and over-produced in order to create a much more sugary and toxic beverage. People became addicted to which is how that industry was able to become so lucrative over the course of the last 100 years or so, give or take a few years.

All of the herbs that were used in the original tonic were a blend of herbs that allowed for a good and solid bowel movement that was a popular way to wake up in the morning and get ready for the day. It is well known that the better, more fashionable way to wake up in the morning at the turn of the 20th Century was with cocaine and not caffeine, and Coca-Cola became an even more potent "herbal remedy" to keep you in high spirits and good health when this ingredient made it into the regular recipe for "Coke".

Many people were addicted to the beverage as a result of its "health benefits" and chose it over other beverages more often, leading to a good deal of altered states at that time, until it was reported that the addictive substance be removed and a new, better addition replace the cocaine: sugar. Little did they know, sugar was just as addictive and somewhat as toxic to the internal rhythms of the human body, leading to a new wave of inspired addictions all over the world.

Each time you pop the cap of a popular soda, or canned sugary drink, remember that it had once derived from a truly powerful healing concoction that was intended to create internal balance and harmony within the body. Not many people know how much work the world has done in order to deny this old knowledge of herbal healing. In the ancient days, you had no other choice: what you see growing in the woods and in the fields is what you get, and so people had to learn how to work with what they had a make a new life with these herbs and how they all had a benefit when used in the right place at the right moment in time.

HERBAL MEDICINE

Today's "herbal market" is acting on a lot of institutionalized ideas about how medicine works and how prescriptions are the answer to all of your health-related problems. In the long history of mankind, the most effective remedies and healing agents have always been and always will be, herbs, plants, flowers, and roots.

No other remedy will bring a full body balance to the system and so it is within the work of your discovery of herbal remedies that you are able to equip yourself with this true and real knowledge about how to manifest the greatest levels of health and inner abundance. When you practice using herbal remedies, you internally balance all of the chemical vibrations within your biology and organ systems in order to create the highest functioning system.

People had no concept of this when herbs were first being utilized; they only saw that there were benefits, results, and curious after effects to some of these uses and were guided by the plants themselves to learn the proper way of being used and when to be used. As we are evolving we have chosen to look less at the benefits of what has already existed on the planet for ages and ages, more at what will make or cost money, and what you trust a doctor will tell you.

As a species, humans have grown into their natural wellness over time through the use of what was available to them. Pharmaceuticals were never a part of that experience when we began to evolve our existence as a thoughtful, intelligent and capable species of critically thinking beings. We never had a need of all of these prescriptions and medical advancements, and to this day, we continue to ruin our health, rather than improve it with all of the advice from medical professionals who believe in the power of drugs to "cure" the sick and weak.

Before questions of this kind began to arise as early as the 1910s, men and women kept all of their faith and beliefs about health in the hands of the doctors and nurses who held the highest knowledge of all matters physical and healthy. News of all of these new remedies and prescriptions were a fashion of the time and the arrogance of doctors, who prescribed their own blends of tonics in order to achieve a greater popularity and interest, beset a new wave of pharmaceuticals that evolved throughout the industry of chemistry and biology in order to manufacture simulations of what herbal remedies were already capable of doing on their own.

All of this was about money and fame and had a lot to do also with curiosity. When we become more knowing about new ideas, concepts, structures of science, beliefs about the body, philosophies about health, then we are naturally willing to try the newest, most obvious and most creative ways of altering our views and ideas of how to heal. "There must be a better way than what we already know, so let's keep looking and researching."

HERBAL MEDICINE

The real truth is that all of these advances in health and science, pharmaceuticals and prescription drugs and even certain surgical procedures, have worked as far away as you can get from the healthiest form of internal body medicine: herbs.

No known drug on the market today has as much benefit in one pill or even a whole bottle as the common ingredient garlic. Garlic has been well known for as long as people have been walking upright and it has always had a major benefit on the whole system in more ways than one. In today's world, it is most often treated as a culinary herb that has a potent aroma and flavor and makes a whole dish an exciting and wonderful treat. There are also a lot of rumors circulating in old folklore that garlic is a good way to keep the vampires away, but let's not open that can of worms.

Garlic is more powerful as a healing remedy than as a cooking ingredient, and the good thing is that if you like garlic in your pasta sauce, then you are making yourself a very healthy dish. Garlic has generally become well known as a potent healer in this world, and it is most often used in this way as a powdered capsule that you swallow with your daily intake of herbal supplements.

The truth of all of that is that although supplements can have a benefit and use to the system, the real healing magic comes from the fresh, dried and chopped up herbs themselves, and not from a processed and manufactured, easy to swallow pill. Garlic has never needed anything to work its magic on the human body system, and as it is digested in your stomach and passes through your digestive system, it releases all of the perfectly wonderful and glorious elements that make it so healing into your body.

Garlic has the power to fight off cancerous growth, prevent illnesses, improve cardiovascular health, promote stamina and weight loss, cure indigestion and bowel issues, kill a variety of harmful bacteria and internal bugs that come and go through our bodies, and so much more. All of the pharmaceuticals on the market are never going to be as glorious a healer as a clove of raw garlic every day and when people return their bodies to the world of herbal healing, they will learn that this type of medicine is, and always will be, the best and most effective manner of taking good care of your health.

The last time you were sick, what did you take? Over the counter nasal and flu medication, or a simple menu of hot herbal teas, herbal nasal steams, garlic, salty broth, and lots of water? Preventing sickness is also a major force of how herbal remedies have worked for thousands of years. When your nutrition is at his highest, you are less likely to become ill and will only need herbs to maintain your health and wellness, and not just for use at the time of sickness.

Herbs are used as a preventive health care system and should always be used in the daily diet to impact overall health maintenance. In the matter of pharmaceuticals, your body actually becomes weaker and less capable of fending of sickness, illness and even serious cases of cancer and disease. These drugs do more harm in the long run then they do good, and it is a long time coming that these concepts of healing will finally result in a return to Nature.

As you read through this book, answer all of your own health questions and concerns through this new lens of knowing about how our culture and society has grown away from the wisdom of herbs and the body and chosen a less healthy path. When you are studying these herbs and how they work, consider them friends of yours who speak a truthful language of well-being and health. You will always have a good friend on your side when you work with the healing power of herbal remedies and as we continue to evolve in our culture and society, more and more people will find their path back to the world of the true healing arts, protecting the whole body with a long and ancient wisdom assigned from the Earth herself.

HERBAL MEDICINE

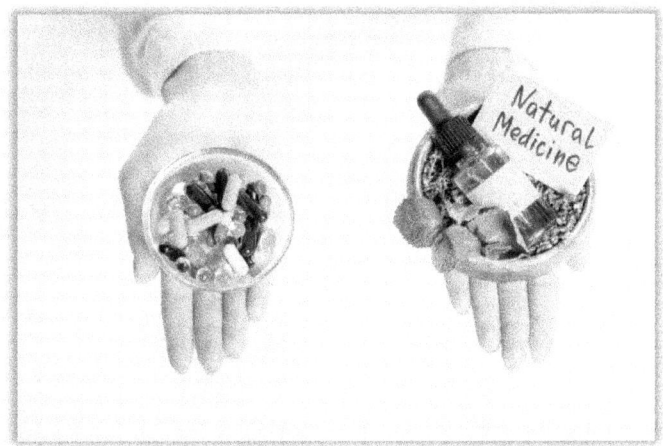

As you go on this journey of knowledge, accept each new method, concoction, remedy and herbal ingredient as a new friend to your budding and growing personal healing practice. Remember the old-world men and women who survived and lived to continue growing and feeding the next generation of life to learn the magic and wisdom of herbs. Protect this knowledge and make it a part of your at-home apothecary while you gain in health, internal wealth, and physical abundance.

CHAPTER 2

HOW TO USE MEDICINAL HERBS

We are all in need of a hot cup of tea on a rainy day or night. We all have a need for a hearty bowl of soup when the weather is cold and when all of us in the family are "under the weather." Practicing with herbal remedies is a good beginning to find ways to bring all of these medicines into your daily life as you gain in confidence with your home healing methods.

All medicine has a time and a place when we are sick and unwell, but how about all of the other times? The importance of using herbal remedies at certain times shows us the best ways of preventing sickness as well as fighting off when it does come to us anyway. The best ways to use medicinal herbs are much more common than you might already be thinking, and there are plenty of ways to use herbs that you are not yet familiar with.

In this day and age, we are all along the road to wellness with our own prescribed notions of health care that came from our childhood experiences with how our parents took care of us when we were ill, and from how doctors and nurses are able to help us with their ideas of prescriptions or pharmaceuticals. The real remedies only need two things to really become useful: water and heat.

All of our hot teas, soups, broths, tonics, hot baths, herbal steams and so on, are the way that most herbs are able to become available to your body system in a quick and efficient manner. Let's talk about how tea has been used for centuries to improve health and give you some pointers as to how all of that knowledge has come into being and why it is still one of the best ways to take medicine today.

Tea has almost always been a part of our human civilizations. As we became a more sophisticated group of people, our ancient ways of "taking tea" were promoted before any other way of healing our bodies. How we came across this tradition was always in many cultures and societies and never started with one person or group; it was innate knowledge that came from a real understanding that when you apply your herb to hot water, it tastes a new way and has a new color. Most people had no idea that they were all collectively creating the best way of healing their bodies and to this day, herbal teas are still heavily used to treat a variety of causes, even just a relaxing and commonly practiced past time: afternoon tea.

The world of tea has become an exaggerated market of heavily produced exotic brands and flavors and they are all just herbs grown in the soil, harvested, dried, processed in facilities, shipped across continents and then dropped into a mug on your kitchen counter where you bring it to life with a kettle of boiling hot water. All the teas in the world are an assortment of herbs and are often colored and flavored as they are processed, if you are utilizing a more generic and less health-conscious brand.

The herbs that you apply to teas could just as easily be grown and harvested from containers in your kitchen window, or garden beds in your back yard and do not need to come in a box to add to your healing cabinet. The best herbs are the ones to tend to yourself and cut down at the right moment to dry and preserve in your kitchen cabinet, preserving the freshness of the herb's true healing power. Not all of us are capable of growing our herbal remedies and require other sources to help us find the best herbs to match our needs. There are plenty of shops around the globe that offer an assortment of semi-fresh cut herbs that you can order, or purchase and add to your cabinet. You can even find a variety of herbs at the local farmer's market that you can bag up, take home, hang upside down and dry for your next batch of at-home herbal remedies.

HERBAL MEDICINE

The only way to give yourself a proper healing dose of herbs, plants, flowers, and roots, is to utilize the elements of water and heat to pull the healing benefits of each plant into the water and then down your throat. The last time you had a cup of herbal tea, was it delicious and soothing? Did it feel warm and beneficial? There are almost always times when you drink something that feels oh so good to your taste buds and body, but there are also those times when you avoid drinking something because it has only bitter or sour tastes.

Those tastes are actually an incredibly vital part of healing and nutrition in the body and a variety of herbs, when made into a hot tea remedy, will produce a strong taste of bitterness, or even hot spiciness, or sourness, that you may not like at all. How can you heal if you don't let all of the ancient wisdom of herbs tickle your taste buds?

Bitterness, sourness, saltiness, spiciness, sweetness and all of the range of taste bud emotions you can imagine are a link to health and herbal medicine that support this reality. Our need to avoid the different tastes comes from a long and addicted journey to sweetness, sugars and salty things, usually preferring these flavors over the other two major ones, bitterness and sourness. All of the flavors are of vital importance to the health of the body and need a good and proper balance to help you align well with your whole health and healing power.

HERBAL MEDICINE

The bitterness factor of certain teas helps your body to ascertain a variety of quality functions, most notably the production of bile to offer a healthier way of digesting food. A long time ago, the most fashionable way, which remains to true to this day, was through the use of what are called aperitifs and digestifs, As a result of all of our needs to enjoy alcoholic beverages with the grand feast, these two beverages were incorporated as a pre and post dinner time drink that would stimulate the body's ability to healthfully receive and digest the meal presented at dinner.

The benefit of these liquor tonics was how they worked well with the body chemistry to stimulate a healthier way of processing and digesting, however, not only was alcohol an unnecessary addition to this quality herbal tonic, it actually ruined the benefit of the herbal ingredients involved in its creation. Without the alcohol, a bitter and slightly sour aperitif, followed by a strongly bitter digestive, wonderfully supports the whole system through the digestive process.

Although these two methods of receiving bitterness and sourness were a common method for receiving quality herbs, they were promoted only as alcoholic drinks after their original worth as an herbal tea remedy.

And now, back to teas. All of the herbs that you read about in this book can be used most effectively as a tea infusion or decoction and as you approach all of these herbs and plants with this knowledge, attempt to find your herbs as a fresh cutting that you will dry on your own at home, or gather them at a local shop that sells herbs in bulk so that you can begin to provide your medicine cabinet with a good assortment of the most classic herbs you will need for your healing journey.

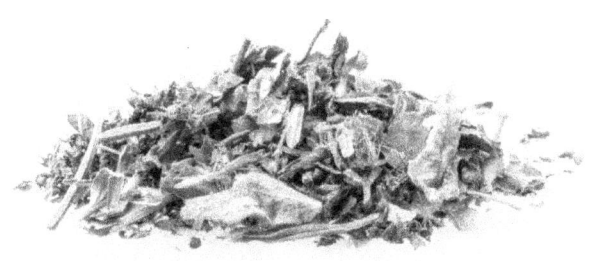

The best way to prepare most, but not all, herbal teas is the following:

The Proper Way to Prepare an Herbal Tea Infusion

1. Gather dried herbs and chop into smaller pieces (if required- not all plants and herbs require chopping or cutting as they can already be small in their leaves and flowers, or naturally crumble after being dried)

2. Bring water to a soft, low boil in the kettle.

3. Pour hot water over loose, dried herbs (you can use a tea strainer to lift the herbs out

before drinking the tea; however a tea ball should be avoided because of how condensed the herbs can get inside the ball, disallowing a full release of all of the plant medicine you are wanting to extract from the herbs)

4. Steep tea for as long as 30 minutes and no less than 10-15 for a fully powerful remedy.

5. Drink immediately. (Avoid refrigerating teas after steeping as they will begin to lose their potency and always best when consumed hot to warm in temperature).

All herbal teas follow a similar method, including flowers stems and leaves, but when it comes to roots, you need to take a different approach. There is a significant amount of healing roots available, either through your own foraging and harvesting, or through an apothecary or teas shop. A majority of these roots are why we have a long-term assessment of health in the first place. A wide variety of cultures and societies have turned to roots to heal the body, and even the hunter-gatherer groups were using them as a way to have food and not because of looking for an herbal remedy, unknowingly incorporating their benefits into their forager's diet.

A root tea needs a different preparation because of the thickness and density of the material you are adding to the heat and water. The best method for preparing a root tea is the following:

The Proper Way to Prepare a Root Tea Decoction

1. Acquire a quantity of dried and/or roasted roots from preferred or needed variety. (Roots are also easily harvested and preserved as well as obtained from local, or online herbal wholesalers and shops)

2. Add the quantity of roots needed for decoction into a small saucepan or simmering pan.

3. Fill a pan with 8-16 ounces of clean water (amount varies depending on the quantity of roots and desired potency of decoction).

4. Bring water and roots added to a boil and then turn all the way down to a low heat to allow for a long and slow simmer.

5. Simmer on low for approximately 10 minutes and remove from heat.

6. Strain and drink.

**NOTE: Because of their potency, you can also reuse the simmered roots for a second batch of tea before discarding them. Although the second round of root tea won't be as potent, it will still contain a large amount of healing benefit.

HERBAL MEDICINE

All of the root teas that you prepare will have a strong and powerful energy of healing because of how a quality of life under the soil, absorbing nutrients, water and minerals over a period of time, causes them to have a thickness of healing power. Having a root tea cabinet in your home healing apothecary is a wonderful way to promote and support continuous good health and healing when fallen ill, or weakened by a variety of causes, including stress, bowel troubles, digestive problems, anxiety, malnutrition, obesity, patterns of light and dark feelings and many more.

Another method of using medicinal herbs, outside of the realm of herbal teas is through the use of soups, broths, and stews. I know what you may be thinking: that is what cooking is, not medicine. However you view the culinary arts, much of how it originally worked was as a way to heal the body as well as feed it. A long time ago, when you ate a bowl of soup or broth, it was usually as a way to cure a sickness, illness, or to recover from a time of being unwell.

The energy of soup, stew or broth has so much power and potency from a medicinal point of view that it will revitalize and revive any and all disasters occurring within the cells of the body. A concoction of several herbs and other vegetables, meats, and bones have a way of calming the entire nervous and digestive systems and assists with the wellness of the whole body, not just one specific area or concern.

A hearty soup is always a good way to incorporate a beneficial herb into your diet to help you cure what ails you, but also as assurance that your immunity is in good balance with your lifestyle and health. A broth on its own is enough to feed and nourish you for an entire day when sipped as meals and should always work its way into the basic diet of any person. None of the pre-made broths that you find at the supermarket have any of the healing qualities of the kind of broth you can make at home with fresh ingredients and herbs.

In a way, broths, soups, and stews are just a more advanced version of a simple, herbal tea, applying the same technique of water and heat to several ingredients to extract their healing benefits to ingest and make you well again. A lot of people prefer the ease and convenience of purchasing boxed or canned soups, stew, and even broths; however, all of these are completely lacking in nutritional quality or healing power.

The way to avoid a soup without any healing benefit is to simply make your own and it as easy as brewing a cup or a pot of tea. Here are the basic instructions for a broth, a soup, and a stew using only a small variety of ingredients:

Basic Broth Recipe

1. Put soup bones, or vegetables, or both into a large pot and add water (coarsely chop the veggies first). Use enough water to at least

cover the bones and add a few extra inches of water to the pot.

2. Add an herbal variety including thyme, rosemary, bay leaves, salt, etc. to the pot.

3. Bring to a boil and skim off any foam that rises to the surface.

4. Turn down to a lower temperature and simmer for approximately 6-8 hours.

5. Strain vegetables and bones from liquid and discard.

6. Refrigerate broth and use daily as an herbal remedy.

Basic Soup Recipe

1. Use your broth from the first basic recipe as a healing base and begin to heat in a pot slowly.

2. Add an assortment of healing vegetables, depending on what your healing needs are and cook to soften. (you can add animal proteins as well and can either cook them in the broth which will add flavor to the soup, or cook separately and add to the soup after the meat is cooked)

3. Add an assortment of healing herbs to flavor the soup and pull out any health benefits from the herbs as you cook, using herbs like basil, rosemary, thyme, bay leaf, pepper, curcumin, celery root, garlic, ginger, and more.

4. Allow all ingredients to cook for at least 1 hour, or more at a low temperature.

5. Use soup immediately for best healing results and reheat as needed.

**NOTE: The longer a soup, broth, or stew is refrigerated, the less beneficial it will be. Always toss a remaining concoction of soup, stew or broth after about 6-7 days in the fridge.

Basic Stew Recipe

1. Use a basic soup recipe to begin your stew, incorporating a thickening agent such as gelatin, or corn starch, but *do not ever use white flour* for a thickening agent as it is very toxic to the body and all of its functions).

2. Add the thickening agent after you simmer your basic soup recipe for about 30 -45 minutes, and allow the thickener to congeal the soup for another 30 -45 minutes of cooking time.

3. Add any extra ingredients you want during cooking, or as the recipe calls for.

4. Salt to taste.

Each of these basic recipes allows you to get a full and powerful dose of medicine from the herbs and plant materials you use, and even some of the animal proteins can add a very strong healing element when purchased from the right farmer, rancher, or butcher.

All soups, stew, and broths use the same basic elements to extract the high quality of healing that exists in all herbs, flowers, roots, plants, and yes, sometimes even animals. The best quality ingredients should always be used and if you can grow them yourself or get them from a local farmer that would be ideal. Organic ingredients are also a better choice than the conventional variety, and all of your herbal ingredients can be easily acquired at the closest grocery store or herbal shop.

Any other kind of soup from a can, a box, the frozen section and so forth, will never be as healing as what you can make in your own kitchen due to processing methods and unhealthy packaging. Most canned soups are not actually made from real or fresh ingredients at all and are just a simulation of what these ingredients would taste like if you actually made it yourself.

There are even more ways that you can use medicinal herbs, and we will go into detail about some, but not all of them. All herbs can be taken and processed by hand and turned into pastes, salves, ointments, tinctures, soaps, scrubs, eye-washes, wound cleaners, extractions, essences, poultices and steams. The next few processes you will learn about will be the easiest and most useful for a beginner, and as you become more advanced in your ability to process herbs in these ways, you can explore the complex and complicated versions of making herbs a useful part of your life.

Basic Salve Recipe

1. Clean and dry fresh herbs of choice.

2. Chop with a knife or in a food processor until fine and small.

3. Melt any of the following: beeswax, shea butter, lard, tallow. **NOTE: you can create a simple blend of all of these or a couple of them together to get the desired texture and consistency. Be sure to use organic and fresh ingredients.)

4. Let the melted fat cool slightly and add your chopped herb to the melted fat agent.

5. Let the herbs sit for a few minutes and then return them to the burner on a low temperature to keep the fat from hardening.

6. Keep at a low temperature for approximately 10 minutes and then remove from heat.

7. Strain the herbs from the fat/ oil blend into a container and either refrigerator or let harden at room temperature.

8. Use as needed.

Basic Essences Recipe

1. All ingredients must be used immediately after harvesting in order for their energy and healing benefit to remain secured in your carrier liquid so be ready to work with your herbs directly after cutting them from your garden.

2. Use pure and clean water, preferably water that has not come from a tap and has not been in a plastic bottle or container.

3. Pour about 1 cup of water into a crystal or glass bowl and place in direct sunlight to warm it up.

4. Trim, cut or puck flowers or herbs from where they are growing, adding only the flower heads

HERBAL MEDICINE

and herb leaves and discarding any stems or roots.

5. Gently place herbs or flowers into a warm bowl of sunlit water while you do something else for a while, at least 2-4 hours for maximum healing benefit to be released into the water.

6. Drain the bowl into a container, allowing the flowers and herb leaves to remain in the water. Make sure the container is a sterile bottle with a lid or a cap that is also sterile.

7. Add a small quantity of alcohol to preserve the essence. Only a little is needed and should be the highest quality you can afford. Use about 1 oz per 1 cup of water. The best alcohol choices are brandy and whiskeys that are well manufactured.

8. Use a small amount, such as a dropper full in a glass of water, twice a day, for the healing energy of the herb or flower used.

9. You can also make a more distilled version of your large water essence and add a small portion of your original essence into a smaller bottle, adding some more water to it. This will create a less potent remedy and will have a

great healing benefit when used over a long period of time.

**NOTE: The reason you would want to distill a base essence with added water is that the flower and herb essence are very strong and can have a more negative impact on your whole system if overused. It is important to understand what ailment you want to treat as you work with essences.

Basic Extraction Recipe

1. Add a large amount of water to a cooking pot and bring to a boil.

2. Add your preferred herbs to the boiling water as you start to simmer the liquid at a lower temperature. Add a large quantity of herbs (more than you would use in a tea) and you can either pick one herb, or use a variety together, depending on what your needs are.

3. Simmer the liquid down until it has lowered significantly in the pot, leaving a smaller amount of liquid than when you started.

4. The remaining liquid should be very dark and potent and will have a strong acidity, or flavor when tasted.

5. Strain herbs from liquid and discard.

6. Use a sterilized container to store the extraction and add a very small quantity of alcohol to preserve the liquid. A general rule of thumb is 1 oz of alcohol to 1 cup of liquid for herbal remedy preservation purposes.

7. Use over the next several weeks as a healing remedy and throw out after about 2 months time if it has not been fully consumed.

All of these basic medicinal preparations are useful for most herbs and flowers and some roots and leaves. Stems are not always used; however, some plant stems can be very healing, depending on what herb you are working with.

So, now that you have some basic understanding of how to use herbal remedies, the question is when. All of your life you have learned from a doctor how to treat your illnesses and ailments and have trusted them to tell you what your illness is and how to treat it. When you are working with herbal remedies, you should use them all of the time, not just when you are ill.

As you have already read, most herbal remedies are used for a preventative measure against sickness and can help you stay well for much longer. At the time of illness, you are usually beginning to notice early signs and symptoms, and this is the perfect time to begin to introduce some of your basic healing recipes into your

HERBAL MEDICINE

daily diet and experience to promote a speedy recovery from a supported immune system and inner balance.

As you are learning to listen to your own body for guidance, you can ask yourself a series of questions to ascertain the best method of healing yourself well. To correlate your needs to each herb, you will work with some of the essential herbs found in other chapters in the book, but for the meantime, look at the list of questions below to help you determine what kind of a remedy you might need for yourself.

- What are my symptoms and are they internal or external?

   If symptoms are internal, teas, soups, broths, extractions, and essences are a better choice than an external salve.

- What is my assessment of my body's energy right now? Hungry? Achy? Feverish? Chilled? Sneezy? Congested? Headaches?
    1. *Hunger: soups, stews, broths, teas*
    2. *Achy: teas, broths, essences, extractions, salves for muscle and joint pain*
    3. *Feverish: Essences and extractions*
    4. *Chilled: Broths, soups, stews, teas*
    5. *Sneezy/Congested: All of the above (make a salve with eucalyptus for the chest and under the nose cavity)*
    6. *Headaches: teas, broths, stews, and extractions*

HERBAL MEDICINE

- When do I feel ill?
  If you are feeling ill at certain times of day it can be related to a number of factors and the best way to assess what herbal remedy you need; you should ask the first two questions listed and answer them.

- What am I trying to heal or prevent and how long will it take for me to work with these herbs to heal or prevent sickness?
  All of your work with herbs has a way of showing you the right method and herbal blend to help you ascertain the best choice for healing. As you learn more about each herb, you will be able to answer this question easily.

- When should I stop using a certain herb to limit an overuse of its healing remedy?
  When you are feeling better from your work with herbs, you can cut way back on what and how you are using your herbal remedy and use it occasionally to support your immune system. Some herbs will be used more often than others on a regular basis, especially culinary herbs and herbal teas.

- Where do I look for the best method of healing myself when symptoms start to arise?
  The answer to this question is as specific as the ailment you are trying to heal, and you will have to work on a case by case basis with all healing and energetic experiences.

Asking yourself a variety of questions about what you want from your herbal remedies will help you find the right one for your purposes. You will never have to worry about overdoing it with a majority of herbs (although some can be toxic in large quantities: see Chapter 7) and you will be able to work with many of them on a regular basis in order to stay healthy and prevent sickness, and also treat illnesses well when they arise.

Whether you are making soups, stew, broths or teas, or you are concocting salves, essences or extractions, each of these methods will help you begin your path to learning and understanding the most beneficial way to use medicinal herbs in your daily life. As you read further, you will learn more about each herb, how to find the best ones, which are the most essential and good for a beginner's medicine cabinet and more recipes to help you explore your healing journey.

CHAPTER 3

SELECTING THE BEST HERBS

Aromatherapy was always a unique tool to help people heal themselves, especially in a time when there was no other way of identifying a scent of an herb or a medicinal value of how it worked well on the human body system. Like all aromatherapy oils and scents, wisdom about herbal remedies follows the lessons of identifying the best ingredients by how they smell.

Many people who work with herbal remedies find out early on that you can quickly tell the difference between an herb, plant, flower, or root that has already turned south and will not be fit for use. A lot of generic brands of herbal remedies found in grocery stores and sold in capsule form utilize herbs that are past their prime in order to consolidate costs and not lose any profits. This is another good reason to support your health by concocting your own herbal remedies so that you are not taking in poor quality medicinal herbs.

The last lesson was all about how to use these herbs and this chapter is going to take a look at how to choose them. When you are looking for the right herbal remedies for yourself it is best to consult a physician about what your symptoms are, however as you gain in trust with yourself and understanding what illnesses you may be prone to, or you are in line with any chronic ailments that need to be regularly treated, then you can discover how to use the herbs in the best way and also how to choose them based on their level of quality.

A lot of people will simply order their herbs from the internet in bulk bags and containers and leave it at that, and while that may be a convenient solution to finding the herbs that you want to use, it is actually a loss to you financially and when you receive the herbs in a bag already harvested and dried, they have lost so much of their healing potency and can sometimes be a lower quality after being harvested too soon or too late.

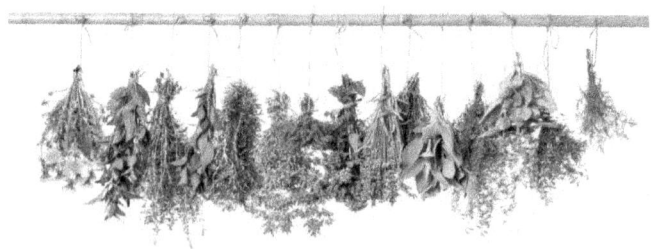

The best way to get your herbs is to grow them yourself, and as that is not always possible for everyone, the next step up would be to locate a local farm or grocer that has a regular supply of fresh herbs or very recently harvest ones. The reason for this is that when an herb is put out on the shelf in a refrigerator, or packaged and dried in a bulk container at the store, its shelf life is already limited to a shorter period of time, resulting in a serious lack of vital medicinal nutrients.

When you are at the grocery store and you are looking in the dried herbs section do you ever ask yourself how long they have been sitting there in their jars or containers? Much of what you find in the bulk section at a supermarket is going to be rancid and no longer fit for human consumption. Anywhere you go this is true, and a lot of people eat a lot of food from the bulk department.

The answer to all of that is to choose fresh ingredients and the best way to find all of those items is at your local farmer's market. When you visit the farmer's market, you can find an array of seasonal herbs and various concoctions to add to your at-home apothecary. You can also ask each farmer that you visit if they ever grow certain herbal items that you may able to purchase in the future. Occasionally, a farmer might be kind enough to start growing some for you, especially if you make a contribution to their market stall regularly.

Another way to get your herbs is to find a local herbal remedy shop that specializes in local herbs, flowers, plants, and roots. These kinds of shops sell herbs out of the jar in bulk so regularly that the chance of getting off, spoiled, or rancid remedies is highly unlikely; however, it's always good to use your nose to check. When in doubt, take a whiff.

The positive side of purchasing your herbs in this way is also that you can develop a close relationship with the shop folks and find out exactly when they refill their jars and containers, or when they get their freshest shipment of goods in stock. You can make a regular appointment with yourself to only go to the apothecary shop on delivery days to ensure that you are getting the best products.

We are all good at knowing when something tastes off, but with herbs, it's always about the smell. Crack open a fresh package of peppermint leaf and take a deep inhale. How does it smell? If all you can smell is peppermint, then it is fresh. If you smell peppermint and a little something extra, then your herbs have gone south, and they shouldn't be used to care for your health.

Much of what you find in the fresh produce section of the grocery store is already on its way out the door in terms of quality, and so looking for a better place to find them will help you immensely with selecting the best herbs for your home medicine cabinet.

Another way of selecting the best herbs for your healing purposes is to use a diagram of registering how long an herb can last after being cut from the source.

HERBAL MEDICINE

You should always take notes and keep your own herbal remedies journal so that you have a way to keep track of all of the lessons you are teaching yourself through the wisdom of herbal medicine.

A chart or diagram of how long an herb lasts after cutting or up-rooting will come in handy as you work with your medicine cabinet. The length of time a sprig of rosemary stays fresh will differ greatly from how long a sprig of thyme will last after being cut.

Drying herbs is a common practice and you should use both fresh and dried herbs regularly to keep a healthy nutritional balance. If you only eat dried herbs, you won't know all of the healing benefits of the plants, and if you only eat the fresh, newly cut herbs, you can cause an excess of gases in the body that can lead to intestinal troubles over time.

Word of warning about asking for a drug store for herbal remedies: all of the alleged "herbal medicines" that you find at the drug store actually have nothing herbal inside of them at all. They are essentially just sugar and pharmaceutical drugs manufactured at a low cost and sold at a high price, marketed as being "herbal." Most people are unaware of this reality and buy into the advertising scheme in the drug and medicine industry. If you truly want to heal yourself, stay away from Big Pharma: it is a one-way ticket to sickness and disease. All you need to do is bring more herbal remedies into your life by selecting the freshest herbs you can find, and sometimes that may mean spending a little extra for the highest quality, but what you save in trips to the doctor's office is well worth it.

CHAPTER 4

ESSENTIAL HERBS

When you are ready to start working with herbal remedies, it is important that you are aware of how each one works with your body and why some are more beneficial than others at certain times in life. Several herbs bare striking resemblance to each other in their actual appearance, taste, and healing properties and so it is important that you look for the right herb or plant for your purposes.

Acquiring a guide book of herbs, plants, and flowers would help you immensely. There is an extensive quantity of various herbs that are used to treat a large variety of ailments and illnesses and so making sure you have the right desk reference of herbs is crucial. Find one that has a picture of the herb as well as a description of how to identify it, where it grows, when it is in season and how to prepare it properly.

Since this book is meant to be a guide for how to treat common ailments with herbal medicines, then you will want to have a companion manual that goes into greater depth and detail about each herb and its uses. One of the most popular ones you can find was actually written in the year 1649 by a man named Nicholas Culpepper called, *The Complete Herbal*.

You may be thinking that something written in 1649 would not be helpful in modern times; however, it is actually more accurate in its assessment of herbal remedies than much of what you can find on the internet or in other books. It is a wonderful beginner's manual and has a lot of information about uses and contraindications, meaning when to avoid using certain herbs, or what parts of herbs to avoid ingesting.

There are a variety of other herbal medicine manuals that can help you. Look for a colorful book that has either photographs of each plant, or herb, or illustrations so that you know what you are looking for. You may want to have more than one herbal dictionary as a reference to help you study and gain the knowledge of each wonderous plant and their gift to you as medicine.

Getting started with herbal remedies is easy when you have the correct application, understanding of its uses and how to choose which one you need and when. All that is needed is the right one at the right moment and here is a short list of some of the essential herbs to keep in your cabinet. Although many of these herbs may already be known to you, it is important that you read each description as a new idea to add to your understanding of these herbs and plants. Keep in mind that as you are reading there will be some information about how you can best utilize each one and why to use them either on a regular basis, or very sporadically to aid in your health and preventative care.

Agaric

Agaric is a fungus, and it looks like a cartoon mushroom from a video game, like Mario Brothers. It has a large red cap with white spots, and although many people have suggested that eating or working with this mushroom will be detrimental to your health, this little, potent remedy will bring you a lot of good health. It has its reputation as being dangerous because it has a lot of look-alikes out there in the forest and so when you are purchasing your agaric from a retailer you won't have any problems because they will have collected the version that will not have a poisonous quality to it; however, if you choose to forage for these powerful babies on your own, make sure you have a mushroom field guide handy or knowledge of the species before you go harvesting.

Agaric has the following health benefits: when prepared the proper way, it aids with indigestions and sparks bowel movement when constipated; gives off a strong and potent amount of acids and chemical compounds that help your immune system build itself up into a greater strength and ability; calms the nervous system; brings a lot of minerals into the diet that are not found in many grocery store foods.

HERBAL MEDICINE

<u>Ways to prepare Agaric</u>: you can dry the caps and store them for later use, rehydrating them with hot water and making a decoction, slowly and low boiling them for around 10-15 minutes to get all of the nutrients out.

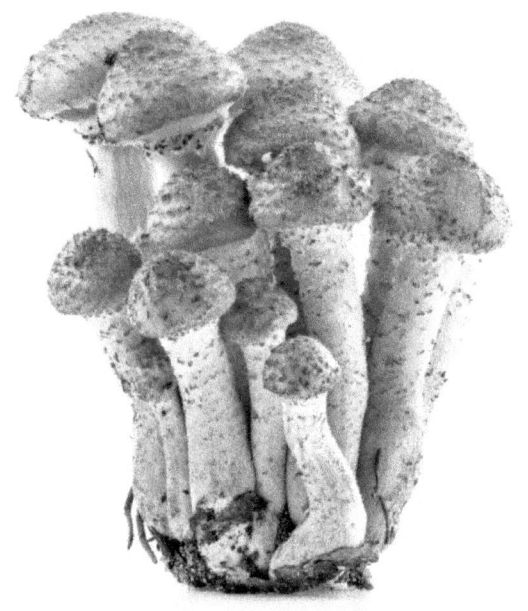

Angelica

Angelica is a sweet little plant and looks a lot like a lover's flower from a lovely bouquet. It has a lot of small white to purple to yellow flowers that when dried are almost along the lines of confetti. The little flowers are the part you will want to use, and they are best used after being hung up to dry while still attached to the stems and leaves. You can hang them upside down in a cool, dry place in your home and hang them above a towel, table, or screen to collect any flowers that fall off during the drying process.

This method can be used for several plants throughout this list and so you can remember it as the **Hanging and Drying Method**. The reason that you will keep the flowers on the stems during drying is that they need all of the moisture they can get during the drying process so that they retain as much of their potency as possible. As the plants are hung upside down, flowers pointing to the floor, all of the moisture in the plant will naturally flow into the petals and remain there the longest, leaving the petals of the flower the last to dry, keeping it the freshest the longest.

Angelica won't take long to dry because the flowers are so small and you can leave some of the leaves on the little flowers as you collect the dried flowers to store them.

Angelica has the following benefits: washes away internal deficiencies when drunk as an infusion of tea; cleanses and purges the system as a detoxifier; blends with all of the other nutrients in the body to create a more harmonious balance and sense of ease with diet and digestion; eliminates problematic bacteria from the digestive system.

Ways to prepare Angelica: the best method is as a tea infusion, however as you become more experienced with these herbal remedies, creating a tincture, an essence, and an extraction would work well long-term for a medicine cabinet.

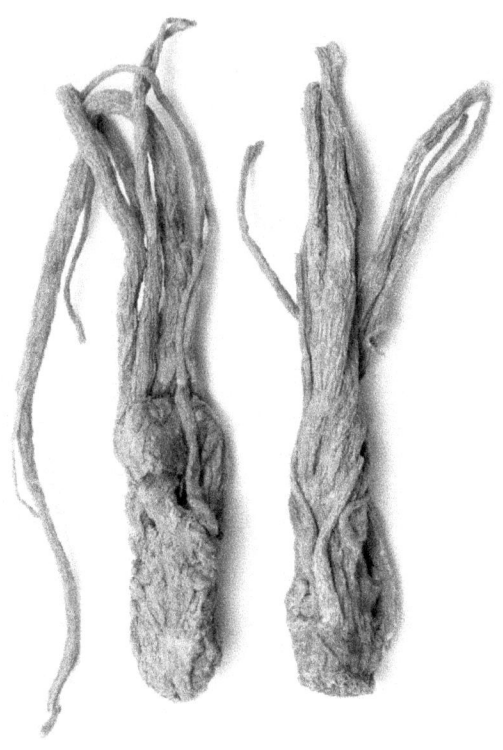

Arnica

Arnica is a dainty little yellow flower, and it grows abundantly all over the place. You may have already seen before in the meadow or park near your home without realizing what it was. Arnica is a very powerful healing agent, especially on the surface of the skin, but internally as well. Many people have used arnica to make salve, ointments, and rubs to soothe aching muscles, stiff joints, tender body parts, and bruises. It has a very strong antiseptic quality as well as a pain killing agent that can help your body work faster to heal all of its sore spots.

Do not use arnica internally if you are pregnant or nursing as a result of it being a strong pain reliever and you will need to have all of your faculties while growing a baby. When you are pregnant and you have pain in your body, you need to discover what the cause is before treating it to be sure that there is no issue with your unborn offspring.

***Note of caution: do not overuse arnica as an internal remedy. It is best used as an external healing herb.

<u>Arnica has the following health benefits</u>: a strong antiseptic and painkilling herb; helps to heal tissues and bruises when sore, strained, bruised, or lacking vital energy.

<u>Ways to prepare Arnica</u>: You can use the salve recipe from Chapter 2, or you can make a simple infusion and sip as a tea. Avoid overuse as an internal remedy as it can become an herb that is overused to relieve pain that doesn't exist anymore. Play it by ear and try one cup a day until symptoms pass and if they don't, ask a doctor.

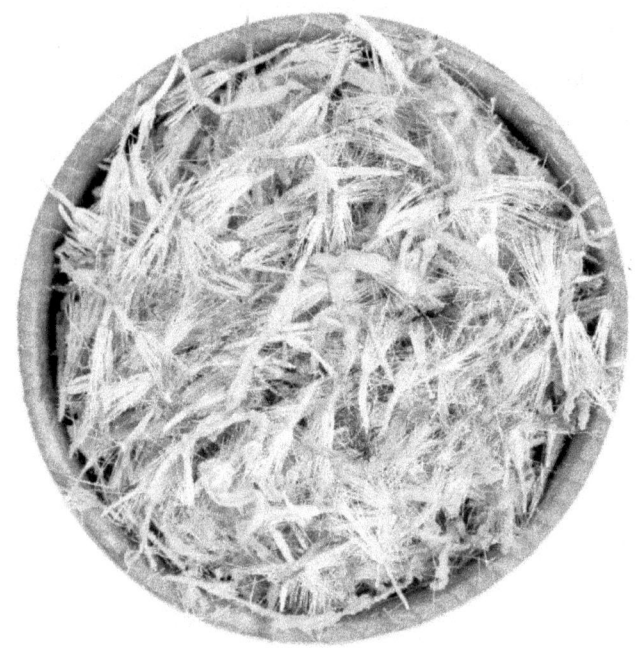

Asparagus

You know asparagus: that long, green vegetable that makes your urine smell funny. It is often eaten as a side dish when it is at its highest volume of growth in the spring. When it has its appearance in the garden, it has a long, tall and fluffy bunch of stems and leaves that feel like a fern or soft hairs and furs. It is quite delicate looking but very sturdy as it grows.

In the herbal medicine process, you will only need these soft, fluffy leaves and stems to create the healing remedy you need to support your health. Although eating the actual vegetable that shoots against these stems and feathers is beneficial to your overall health, in order to receive the true gift of the plants power you will need to harvest the feathery leaves from the bushel.

Asparagus has the following health benefits: Asparagus will act as a diuretic on your urinary system as well as help you cleanse any toxicity in your liver. The way it eliminates these toxins is through the urine, and so it can be a very useful cleansing herb when you are in need of a detox.

Ways to prepare Asparagus: when you dry the leaves and stems to store them, you can then make an herbal tea infusion with the dried materials, and this is the most useful method for utilizing this herb. Much of the flavors will be reminiscent of the beloved vegetable and so you will have a known sense of taste with this one. No other method will act as well as an infusion, so try not to work with any other preparations on this delicate plant. You can brew an infusion and add the liquid to a cleansing or detoxifying smoothie as well.

Barley

Barley, as you may know, is a very popular grain and is often used for cooking in soups and stews and has a very filling quality. It has also been known as a supplement to wheat, which grows in a similar fashion and produces a small grain seed and hull that is processed for bread, flours and other wheat products.

Unfortunately, over time the processing of these grains has stripped them of their nutrient values and they are now more harmful than good to the human body. Wheat especially has been marketed for a long time as the best grain to use for everything, and while that works itself into so many worlds of eating and all cultures of diet, the fact of the matter is that wheat causes a significant amount of dietary dysfunction due to poor growing methods and over harvest and processing.

Barley has also seen its fair share of poor quality growing and harvesting methods, and so you will want to be careful how you choose your source of this medicinal herb. The best way to find high-quality barley is to plant a small patch of it in your landscaped gardens at your home, but if that is not possible, ask your local farmer for freshly sown barley for your stores.

<u>Barley has the following health benefits</u>: digestive aid; balances pH level in the blood and is also a blood purifier and detoxifying agent; eliminates poisons from the body; cleanses the bowels; drives out harmful agents and bacteria; blends well with other herbs to make a powerful health tonic and is a good base for tonics like that.

<u>Ways to prepare Barley</u>: Barley is a grain and so making an infusion or decoction isn't really going to work. The best way to extract the essential medicinal properties of barley is by simply soaking the grain pearls in water

overnight. Water is the agent that will pull all of the minerals and healing compounds out of the tough little grains and so all they need is a little time to soak in this liquid agent. You will want to use a sterile, glass jar that has a lid so that you can cover the soaking grains and always be sure to rinse the grains for several minutes in warm water before starting the soaking process. You can simply drink the liquid on its own, or you can use it as a base liquid for making other concoctions and tonics. Working with barley on a regular basis is an incredibly healthy way to support your body's immunity and general well-being.

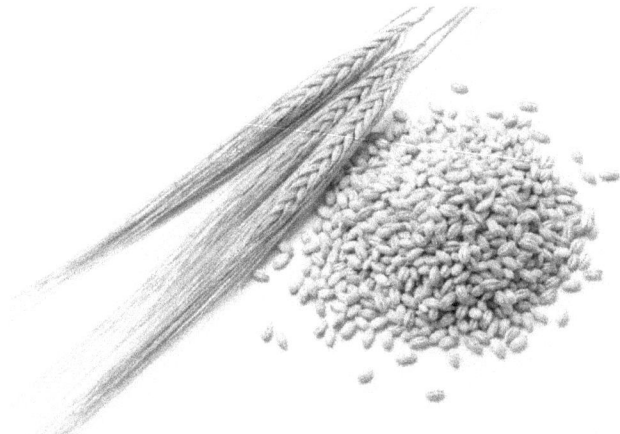

Basil

Basil is a sweet and delicious herb that is easy to grow in any garden. Even an indoor garden would be a good place to grow basil and keeping some around your house is always a good choice. Basil is a well known and popular culinary herb and is most often used to

HERBAL MEDICINE

flavor world-wide dishes and isn't considered regularly for its healing benefits; however, it has a potent taste but also a potent medicine for your health and well-being.

Basil grows quickly and easily in direct sunlight and is always a thirsty little plant. The leaves are where the magic lies and so when you are harvesting your basil, the leaves are all you want to take from the plant so that it can continue to produce more leaves for you. As you are working with the basil leaves, you will notice their powerful aroma and their sweetness of taste. They are both earthy and sweet and bring a powerful flavor to any dish when chopped and sautéed with your noodles or sprinkled over your eggs. Even just cooking with this delightful herb brings a benefit to your diet and so it has its biggest health potency when made as an infusion, an essence, extraction, or even just chewed fresh and eaten like a snack.

<u>Basil has the following health benefits</u>: Detoxifier of the blood; supports a healthy liver and gallbladder; greases the wheels of all of your internal organs; packs a huge load of nutrients and minerals to help with cellular functions; deposits appropriate amount of vital nutrients into the places starved of them, such as in certain organ or cellular systems; awakens the nervous system and soothes the nerves; calms the actions of the nervous system and brings a sense of relaxation.

<u>Ways to prepare Basil</u>: eat it raw and fresh- added to meals, taken as a snack to chew on, chopped and

sprinkled onto dishes for flavor; use fresh or dried herbs as an herbal tea; make an essence or extraction.

Blackberry

Blackberry is a well-known invasive species of thorny berry bush and has its whole healing property in the berry. Blackberries are a vital mineral and nutrient-rich food and have a majority of their power in the sweet, juicy, pudgy little fruits that are produced from the delightful flowers that bud open in the spring. By the summertime, blackberries are ready for harvest and can be eaten directly off the bush to provide you with their healing powers. The juice of the blackberry is powerful and can heal almost any cough you may have and will always be useful during times of congestion or abnormalities in breathing and bronchial issues.

The leaves of the blackberry bush, as well as the flowers, are not as often available at the right moment for healing the body and so when you are looking for health remedies, only use the berry for the purpose of potency. Although the flowers will make a beneficial herbal essence and the leaves can make a hearty infusion of tea, the best choice for optimal health is to use the berries only. Avoid purchasing conventional berries because the last thing you want on your healing path is a whole lot of chemicals sprayed on the berries and then consumed when you eat them. This is very poisonous to the health of your whole system. Instead, look for places along the highway, or throughout the neighborhood for a big overgrowth of blackberry bushes. As I said, it's an invasive plant and will grow quickly all over the place, and so eventually you will come by it in the area where you live. Picking the fresh berries is the best way to bring them into your medicine cabinet.

<u>Blackberry has the following health benefits</u>: Aids in the relief of coughs and colds; brings a lot of healing remedy to the lungs and bronchial tubes; supports a healthy lung immunity; heals sinus problems as well as joint inflammation and tissue repair in the ligaments and connective tissues in the body; opens up all of the blood vessels to receive a healthier blood flow; cardiovascular health; cancer prevention.

<u>Ways to prepare Blackberry</u>: Take only fresh berries for processing; eat right off of the bush and limit quantity to when you are full and don't overeat with these because of their high sugar content; you can cook them down and make a syrup for coughs and colds; press them to make a fresh juice.

Borage

Borage is a lovely little plant with blue-purple flowers that look like stars, causing some folks to call this little plant, starflower. It has a fuzzy softness on both the flowers and the leaves and stems, and each plant packs a potent energy and healing quality for your home medicine cabinet. Although this little flowering plant has been accused in the past of being harmful or toxic when used in large quantities, nothing could be farther than the truth, and this mistake comes from a lack of understanding other health concerns that are volatile and do not properly function with the use of certain herbs. Some of these health concerns include diabetes, rheumatoid arthritis, irritable bowel syndrome, joint pain, muscle spasms, and headaches.

On the other hand, when you are using borage with your problems of the heart, kidneys, gallbladder, and lungs, you will find a lot of powerful health benefits. The reason you want to carefully avoid using borage when you are dealing with any of the above health concerns is that it has an acidity level that requires a more balanced system in order to be well received. Certain ailments have a powerful reaction to high acid levels, and so when you are trying to find the right herbs for your healing journey, you will need to have a clear understanding about your personal health at the present moment. A cause of the issue with selecting borage for your remedies has to do with looking at what ideas you have about how you are needing to heal which is why being very open to listening to your body's needs is a key ingredient to working well with herbal wisdom. Your intuition can be a powerful ally in this process; however, you may need to get a physical exam every once in a while to ask your doctor how your levels are in all of your systems. When you are in a balance with your whole body, you will be better equipped to handle each ailment as they come, or provide the proper preventive care for your lifestyle and well-being.

<u>Borage has the following health benefits</u>: detoxes a variety of systems including the kidneys, gallbladder, lungs and chest area, heart cavities and blood; provides an essential nutrient and mineral compound balance to aid in the relaxation of involuntary muscle responses to allow for a healthier function; delivers a potent and long-lasting energetic remedy to the health of the heart and lungs to help with the mucous production of the lungs and the bronchial tubes and the health of the cardiac muscles for optimal pumping and blood flow.

<u>Ways to prepare Borage</u>: the flowers are the only part of the plant that you will need to concern yourself with at this time, however as you become more advanced in your herbal medicine studies, you can include more of the leaves and stems into your work with its healing benefits. The flowers should be kept fresh and never dried because with these little babies all of the potent magic of the herb is lost when cut and dried, so you will want to prepare your kitchen or apothecary are to receive the flowers for preparation before you harvest them for medicinal purposes. The best way to use these flowers is to make an essence. The essence of the borage flower is a well-known remedy with the Bach Flower Remedies system and has been notable as a healer of all of the above-listed issues and ailments. Do not process these flowers in any other way as it will result in a lack of healing power, or will overcook the plant and make it a toxic ingredient in your pantry.

HERBAL MEDICINE

<u>Burdock</u>

Burdock is an elegant looking weed that grows all over the place and has been known to have influenced the invention of Velcro. The burrs of this weed are easily stuck to the fur of an animal walking by, and as a result, the seeds are then carried away to another place on the backs of animals and land in a new area to start to grow and are incredibly fast growing. The burrs themselves are not useful for healing purposes, but the leaves and the roots are very powerful as a health remedy.

The leaves are often used to support a variety of ailments and are usually dried and stored to make an infusion or an extraction. The roots are where the best medicine lies and digging the roots out of the ground can be a challenge because of how deep the dig into the Earth to find nutrients in the soil. The roots when harvested are what gives you the longest lasting benefit and will always be kept well when dries first. The best way to prepare the roots is by washing them cutting them into 1/3 inch round slices, laying them on a baking sheet and slowly dehydrating them at a very low temperature. Degrees and cooking times can vary from oven to oven and the most general time/temperature ratio would be 45 minutes/ 200 degrees F. Once you have dehydrated the roots you can seal them in a container to keep them fresh and use as needed.

<u>Burdock has the following health benefits</u>: respiratory health; healing low back pain caused by kidney toxicity; aggressive diuretic to release all toxins from the body;

muscle and joint health; positive source of minerals and vitamins.

Ways to prepare Burdock: using the dried leaves you can make an herbal tea, or you can prepare an extraction using the instructions from Chapter 2. For the roots, you will use a decoction method and the instructions can also be found in Chapter 2. There is an even yummier way to enjoy the roots after they are harvested, cleaned and sliced. Instead of dehydrating them until all of the liquids have left them, you can also sauté the freshly sliced rounds in butter with garlic and mushrooms and some other fresh herbs and just eat the roots like a side dish with your daily meals. They are very nutritious when eaten and have an equal amount of healing benefit when cooked an eaten in this way.

Chamomile

Chamomile is a very well-known herb and has popularity in many over the counter drug stores and medicinal herbal shops. It has a way of soothing you and relaxing you to the point of sleepiness, and so it is often used as an herb to aid in relaxation and sleep disorders, as well as anxiety, depression, panic attacks, paranoia and other mental health and emotional disturbances.

The best way to use chamomile is through drinking it like a tea as the ritual of the hot beverage in the warm cup sipped slowly over time adds to the benefit of a relaxation meditation you may need to do in order to calm the nerves. The health benefits of this herb do not stop there, and as you read further, you just might be surprised at all of the new ways you didn't know chamomile can aid in the whole health of your body.

<u>Chamomile has the following health benefits:</u> supports healthy sleep and relaxation; clams the mind and body; relaxes muscles, joints, tissues and nervous system functions; offers a potent dose of vitamins and minerals in the form of chemical compounds that release through the digestive system; unclogs arteries in the heart; brings out all of the elements of toxic gases in the body to be cleanly released in the form of flatulence; eliminates all need for any pharmaceutical drugs that are used to calm the nerves or support relaxation.

<u>Ways to prepare Chamomile Tea</u>: Just drink tea made from the dried flowers, and that's all you need to do.

Comfrey

Comfrey has a powerful way of healing wounds and should mostly only work with topical treatments for your herbal healing remedies. The reason for this is that when comfrey is ingested in any quantity, it can transform all of the energy of your lymphatic system into a difficult flow. Because your lymph system has to flow in order to process and release toxic compounds and elements, comfrey has a negative side effect on the internal level and will only be helpful on the surface.

In order to harvest the comfrey plant, all you need to do is pluck the flowers and take a small portion of the leaves from the plant and blend the two together for your medicine making practices. The flowers and leaves will work well dried or fresh and will actually become more potent in the drying process, so it will depend on what level of medicinal strength you are looking for.

<u>Comfrey has the following health benefits</u>: as an astringent when made into an infusion or essence; as a salve to treat and heal scabbed wounds, stitches, scrapes, scars, insect bites and can also be used as a repellent for insect bites, stings, and other external wounds of the skin.

<u>Ways to prepare Comfrey</u>: To prepare the flowers as an astringent, follow the instructions for making a tea infusion or an essence in Chapter 2; to make a comfrey salve, follow the instructions for that application in Chapter 2. Use only topically unless otherwise indicated by your herbal medicine studies.

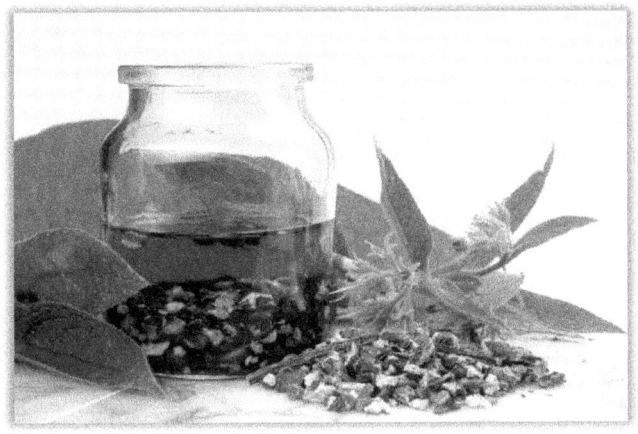

Dandelion

You see them all over the place in the Spring and Summer months of the year: yellow dandelion flowers and their seeds that look like an orb of white lace ready to be blown in all direction, also known as "the wishing flower." Dandelion has all of its benefit in the roots and leaves and not in the flowers and seeds, and the best choice for your health cabinet is to use these parts of the plant for healing purposes.

The leaves are best taken in as food and can be added to any garden salad or can be sautéed in butter or olive oil as a side of bitter greens. The roots are where you find the most potent healing remedy, and when you are preparing the roots for your healing purposes, you will consider them like you are cutting wood chips and bark from a tree because they are tough to chop. The roots, like the burdock, should be washed and dehydrated at a low temperature in the oven or dehydrating machine for a slow drying method so that they can retain all of their healing properties without cooking them out. The longer the better with these little tough roots and the dryness matters when storing them. They will mold if any moisture is left inside and because it is better to roast them first and then cut them, you may have to take and sample root to cut it in half and see if it looks fully dried on the inside.

The dried roots are left to cool for at least an hour before you start to chop them up and I would recommend a food processor if you have one to pulverize the roots into smaller pieces for storage. The best way to store the roots is in a cool, dry, dark area so that they can retain their potency and healthy vigor.

<u>Dandelion has the following health benefits</u>: The leaves when eaten raw or cooked help with aiding digestion of foods and production of bile from the gallbladder which helps break down fats and proteins more efficiently. The leaves are also a great way to eliminate waste from the body as they act as a diuretic and stool softener, so if constipation is an issue for you, try some fresh or cooked dandelion greens. The roots area powerful and healthy package of vital nutrients, mineral, and vitamins and when consumed daily will help your body remain in good health. The roots have a powerful diuretic quality like the leaves and also work as a powerful liver cleansing potion that will keep your liver in good condition and high function. There are a lot of ways too that these roots can stimulate hair and nail growth as well as cell

regeneration of the skin cells. This will be a healthy way for you to enjoy bright eyes and skin and strong, shiny hair and nails. Cosmetically, dandelion root will keep you looking young and ageless if used on a regular, or daily basis.

<u>Ways to prepare Dandelion</u>: harvest fresh leaves, wash and either add to salads or make a side dish with onions, garlic leeks olive oil and add a dash of salt and a crack of pepper- sauté. With the roots, after proper drying and chopping you can make a root decoction by simmering the roots (see instructions in Chapter 2). Drink a few cups every day for optimal health.

Dill

Dill weed has been grown in almost every herbal garden since humans knew how to farm for their food. The dill plant has a soft, feathery leaf and has a portion of its tops that turn to a yellow explosion of buds that look like a firework going off in the sky. The flower part of the dill plant, although lovely, does not contain the richest healing benefits and so it is the leaf and stem of the plant that is most often utilized. A famous culinary herb, the dill weed is used to flavor pickles, most notably, as well as a variety of other dishes. Some cultures prepare nearly every meal with dill and consider it the most nutritious herb on Earth. The Scandinavian diet is one that will use dill on a daily basis for multiple meals, and the health of that culture has been notable for many generations of people.

Dill has a soft, light, and spring-like flavor and aroma and it is a very powerful healing agent for the processes of all of the body systems, but most especially in the work of the spleen, kidneys, pancreas, and gallbladder. These organs are always working so diligently to keep your body in a high functioning state, and when you add dill to your diet, you are offering these organs the chemical and nutrient support they need to stay balanced and healthy.

Dill has the following health benefits: promotes the release of toxins from the spleen, kidneys, pancreas and gallbladder; cures indigestion; opens the arteries, skims off the top layer of fat from your eating, for example a very buttery dish when complimented with dill has a better health benefit for your body as the dill works well with the fat to be better processed by the body, helping the fay offer a more significant nutritional value to your system; protects against diseases like cancer and chronic problems of the kidneys, liver, spleen, and digestive system.

Ways to prepare Dill: eat freshly cut from the garden as an addition to all possible dishes you enjoy dill with- some include eggs, potatoes, salads, vegetable side dishes, soups for flavor or as a garnish on top.

Elder

Elder is a large tree-like bush that can grow to be a rather tall plant in your garden, so you will need plenty of room for it to get larger. The elder plant has a significantly healing property in all of its flowers, berries and yes, even the leaves, bark and roots, although the roots are rarely used in order to preserve the life of the large plant and foster the seasonal growth of generations of healing power. The most effective remedy for coughs and cold in the herbal medicine cabinet is the elder plant, and it is usually the flowers and berries that are used for this remedy. You can use the bark and leaves for these same purposes, but for the simple instructions of a beginner herbalist, we will only discuss the preparations with the flowers and the berries.

<u>Elder has the following health benefits:</u> promotes a healthy immune system; aids in the relief of coughs, colds and sinus problems and infections; works well on a sore throat when gargled; is a powerful concoction when made into a syrup for healing any common cold and can even protect the body during cold season against getting colds; purifies the blood and the arterial walls of the heart; decongests the lungs and helps expel phlegm from the body.

<u>Ways to prepare Elder</u>: you can use the dried flowers only to make an herbal tea to drink multiple times a day during onset of cold and flu-like symptoms and drink regularly as part of your preventive health care program; the berries can be processed into a syrup by heating them in water to release their healing benefits from the berry, like a decoction (instructions in Chapter 5). The berries should not be eaten raw as they can cause an upset stomach due to some of the chemical compounds that need to be cooked down

HERBAL MEDICINE

with heat and liquid. You can also combine the flowers and berries when concocting your herbal elder syrup for a bigger healing potency.

Garlic

Garlic is the master herb, and no medicine cabinet or kitchen should be without it. When in doubt, use garlic. It has a long history of being cut up and expressed to release the juices to heal wounds, warts, liver complaints, flatulence, dysentery, cancerous growths, diseases of the lungs, heart and vital digestive organs, and so many more treatment varieties. Garlic will never go out of fashion as a culinary herb because of how powerful and delicious it can be when cooked to flavor all kinds of dishes and once it enters your body it already had a way of controlling your levels of blood sugar, promoting a healthy level of insulin production and as a result can be a very useful remedy for people who already have, or are in danger of diabetes. The best way to use garlic is by ingesting it and all of the powerful and potent healing properties in each clove will align your body in a healthier way as a prevention of illness, disease and various other conditions. Don't be afraid to use a lot of garlic as it has some of the most beneficial healing power you will find in all of the herbs in this book and many others.

Garlic has the following health benefits: can reduce inflammation in the muscles, bones and joints; has a protective power against many health issues and is even a powerful antifungal, antiseptic and anticoagulant of the blood and lymph as well as other fluids in the body; protects against the power of fecal diseases like IBS, gastroenteritis, diverticulosis, diverticulitis, and colitis; releases a beautiful array of acids and minerals into the bloodstream to help purify the blood in all of the body as well as help to flush any toxins from the body; brings around the aging process and slows it down to a healthy level, keeping you young and fresh in body and mind; promotes a long life-span; works against cancerous cells to protect the body and fight cancer from growing into an unmanageable state; delivers a nutrient power package to all of your organs and tissues; destroys harmful bacteria.

Ways to prepare Garlic: Eat it daily in every meal you can comfortably enjoy it in and don't be afraid of a little garlic breath. You can also make a decoction by simmering cut cloves in water for 10-15 minutes to make a garlic liquid to drink at a meal or after a meal. Garlic can be added to almost any broth, soup or stew and should be if you also want the added benefit of the powerful flavor.

Ginger

This lovely little root produces a gorgeous, tropical looking flower that when you sniff it, it smells like the famous root that has been used for ages to treat a long range of ailments and symptoms. Ginger has a notorious reputation for calming the stomach, especially when feeling nauseated, and will always be a good ingredient to keep in the kitchen to flavor certain dishes and meals.

Garlic is a world-renowned remedy for its ability to calm the intestinal tract, and what it can also do for you is clear away any harmful bacteria and internal issues of the digestive system like intestinal worms, candida (with the removal of sugar from the diet), irritable bowel syndrome, and gastroenteritis. Ginger was also a good friend of garlic in the herbal remedies practice of long ago as the two together pack a very powerful healing punch, no matter what you are suffering from. Together they are the perfect cold and flu tonic and should be used often during times of sickness.

Ginger has the following health benefits: aids in the health of the digestive system; kills bacteria and other harmful entities; soothes nausea; treats problems of the intestinal tract like candida, after sugar is removed from the diet; plays an important role in overall immunity to illnesses.

Ways to prepare Ginger: you can cook with ginger, adding it to a variety of dishes, soups, broths, and stews; you can make a simple decoction with the ginger and drink it as a tea (adding garlic adds an even heftier healing power and benefit); you can also eat it or swallow it raw in small pieces. Cut a pill-sized piece of ginger and swallow it with some water to aid with nausea.

HERBAL MEDICINE

Honeysuckle

Honeysuckle is a well-known flowering shrub, and it has a very sweet and powerfully honey like aroma when the flowers are open and in bloom. The honeysuckle flower is the only healing herb we will talk about in this compendium, but you can research application s for using the leaves and stems from the bush for healing benefits. The flowers are edible, and you can simply pluck them and chew them like a sweet little flower candy, but you will want to limit the quantity that you eat in this way because they can produce a feeling of nausea when over-eaten.

Honeysuckle has the following health benefits: protects against Lyme disease; filters toxins from the blood; produces an amount of lectin for the body that may benefit an ability to control your immunity and fight against diseases like intestinal worms, bowel diseases, as well as other issues like circulation, broken capillaries on the face, muscle spasms and cramping and anything having to do with the lymphatic system and its ability to drain well.

How to prepare Honeysuckle: Eat the raw flowers right off of the branches or garnish your fresh salad with them. Be sure only to pick the freshest blossoms. If they look dry anywhere, you don't want to use them for eating and digesting. You can also collect the fresh blossoms in order to make a flower essence and then you can take a diluted form of it on a daily basis for a short period of time while you heal your ailment that calls for this flower. Teas are an acceptable form of ingestion. The blossoms will need to be harvested and scattered across a screen so that they can dry out. You can make your own drying screen or buy one. It is basically the same material used to screen a window, but you would just make a square or rectangular wooden frame to attach the screen to and lay it down over a barrel or in a way that keeps a good airflow underneath the screen. You don't want to lay it down on a counter or table top because air needs to circulate around the blossoms as they sit on top of the screen. Dried flowers can then be stored and kept in sterile mason jars in a dark, cool place and will then make a sweet and delicious tea when made as an infusion.

Lavender

Lavender is a delightfully aromatic herb that is even a relaxing plant to look at because of its color. The lavender herb plant has had a variety of uses for a while but has also lost some of its traditional medicinal understanding due to modern publications about what this plant can be used for outside of relaxation, calmness, sleep aid, and anxiety or depression issues.

All lavender has the same powerful healing ability, and so it doesn't matter what variety you are using. The only part of the plant that you will need to worry about ever is the flower. The stems and leaves have no real healing benefit or nutrient value so you will not need to harvest these parts of the plants when building your home apothecary. The flower is well planted in any garden or herbal potted plant space you may have and grows well in a variety of soils and conditions however it does not enjoy being overly wet in the roots so make sure you don't over water it if you are growing your own at home.

<u>Lavender has the following health benefits</u>: relaxes the nervous system; depresses the adrenal glands along the ways of pushing them back into a balanced functioning mode (too much caffeine and stressful lifestyle can cause adrenal fatigue and lavender aids in rebalancing these glands so that they can function properly); dries out oils in the skin when applied as an astringent or an essence; performs as a detoxifier when consumed as an edible flower on top of salads or other delicious homemade treats; balances the pH of the body; delivers a huge potency of lectin into the bloodstream which helps to relieve a lot of muscle cramps and spasms, but also helps to relax the muscles in general.

<u>Ways to prepare Lavender</u>: The flowers can be cut and dried for later uses, or they may be used as a fresh herb for floral remedies like essences or infusions. Extractions are trickier with this lovely and soothing herb, so sticking to dried or fresh herbal teas, essences, steams, and salves will be the most appropriate choice for this floral herb.

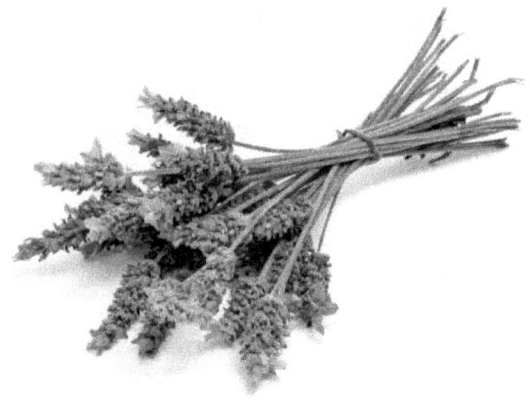

Mint

The most commonly used herb to freshen the breath, mint is a well-known herb that tickles the taste buds and refreshes the mouth and it has a lot of other valuable and medicinal properties. The mint plant has a lot of varieties, and each of them has a medicinal contribution to the systems of the body. The plant leaves and stems are both used in herbal teas and other concoctions, and you will almost never use the roots or flowers of this plant, although the flowers are not harmful and can be eaten; they just don't pack the same punch as the leaves and stems do.

Mint will always be advisable in the case of digestive aid and also contains a variety of other purposes less well known. The mint leaf has a strong ability to loosen the stool when there is an issue of constipation. It can also have an impact on the mucous production that helps all areas of the body that need a healthy supply of mucous. We are never really sure how well our

HERBAL MEDICINE

mucous membranes are working, and so it is a good idea to just support them with a daily or weekly dose of mint in the diet or beverage intake. The best way to enjoy mint is by making a tea infusion, but you can also chew it in the mouth and swallow it in small quantities.

<u>Mint has the following health benefits</u>: aids in digestion and promotes fragrant breath; develops mucous in membranes throughout the body; helps with constipation by loosening stool; as a tea infusion or as an essence it can also be used to aid with specific gastrointestinal disorders over long stretches of time.

<u>Ways to prepare mint</u>: tea infusions and essences. When making a tea you can use both fresh cut and dried mint leaves and stems, but with the essences, you will want to use leaf and flower only during a preparation.

Mugwort

Mugwort has been used for a long time as the witch's herb to relieve all of the issues of warts, skin conditions, diarrhea, kidney stones, gallbladder abnormalities, liver toxicity, dementia, cholic, fungal infections both internally and externally, and a lot more! Mugwort was always a common herb because of how many useful purposes it has and will always be a valuable resource in your medicine cabinet. It is a curious looking little plant and has a lot of low-lying leaves and pretty little flowers that dip down at the top of their stems.

The Mugwort leaves, flowers, stems, and roots are all beneficial and should all be considered for harvest or purchase when you are building your at-home apothecary. The less of it you use, the better because even though its healing benefits surpass many other herbs, it can be toxic if overused in quantity. Making your Mugwort work for you means letting it decide how long you need it; you will get an idea if you are overusing it because your stool will look black and loose after too much use. The less you use at each ingestion, the easier it is for your body to use it well because a little goes a long way and you will only need a teaspoon or two of the dried herbs to benefit from its magic.

<u>Mugwort has the following health benefits</u>: helps remove warts when applied externally and take internally; helps clear and heal several kinds of skin conditions when applied externally as a salve and internally as a tea; helps aid with problems of the colon and large intestine relating to cases of diarrhea; loosens kidney stones and helps break them up into smaller pieces that are easier to pass through the urinary tract; cleanses and purifies the gallbladder; cleanses and purifies the liver; aids with a lot of mental health disorders and diseases including dementia, Alzheimer's, Parkinson's, and others; purifies lung congestion and possible cholic problems by promoting a better opening for the lungs through the process of dilation; cures and relieves the system of internal and external fungal infections; protects the body by

strengthening immunity; allows for a higher performance of work with the digestive system and prevents diseases of the intestines, colon, and stomach.

Ways to prepare Mugwort: As a tea, you can utilize all parts of the plant through the use of dried leaves and/or flowers with or without the use of the root which can be brewed on its own as a decoction.

Mullein

Mullein has an essential quality of removing mucus from the lungs as either a smoked herb or as a tea. The plant itself has very low, broad leaves that are soft and hairy that actually have antifungal properties and the Native Americans used these large leaves to tie to the bottoms of their feet as shoes and to help with any foot problems including wounds and infections. The leaf od the plant is not used for the lungs and remains effective only for external uses, as described by the Native American's use of them.

The tall, long stalk is very thick and sturdy and can reach over 6 feet tall. The top of the plant has a large cob of flowers that can be harvested and dried, and when the flowers are dried, they are very soft, fluffy and thick and work well as a tea infusion or rolled up as a smoke, and even smoked through a pipe. The reason you would smoke the herb is to help expel any clogs in the lungs as it is an expectorant and the smoke help to heal the lungs as you breathe in the herb. Not all herbs can be smoked, and smoking is not recommended to anyone who has serious or chronic

HERBAL MEDICINE

lung disorders or diseases such as emphysema or asthma. When sipped as a tea, Mullein can provide the same support as an expectorant and lung cleansing agent and so if smoking this herb is not a viable option for you tea will work just as well, though you will have to consume it more frequently to help you clear your lungs out.

<u>Mullein has the following health benefits</u>: promotes lung health; clears out lung congestion; improves ability to take deep breaths through the opening of the bronchioles and alveoli; acts as a powerful expectorant when smoked or consumed as a tea infusion; the leaves can be used to help heal wounds and also act as a powerfully useful external antifungal; opens the nasal cavities and all air passages to receive more oxygen through the breath.

<u>Ways to prepare Mullein</u>: Harvest and dry flowers and store in a sterile mason jar and use the dried herbs for herbal teas that can be regularly drunk and also smoked to help heal lung ailments (word of caution about smoking Mullein: you don't need to do it several times per day while healing yourself; once a day is plenty until symptoms are relieved. Too much smoke is also very damaging, so be mindful and alternate between smoke and tea). For external health using the large, fuzzy leaves, you can take a fresh cut leaf and bind it to a wound or infection with twins or string while it heals, but you can also chop it up and make a poultice which just requires the chopped herb and a small amount of cooking fat to make a paste. You can

also use castor oil or other oils that your skin accepts to make it a stickier paste. Apply the paste to the wound or sore and then cover it with a whole Mullein leaf. If it is an open wound that needs medical attention, see a doctor first for care and then use Mullein to help your wound heal more quickly.

Nettle

Nettle, also known as Stinging Nettle, has its name for a reason. The herb, as it grows, develops sticky stinging hair-like barbs that exude a chemical that when touched by your skin cause an irritation that feels like burning or stinging; its almost getting stung by many teeny tiny little bees at once. Although the stinging nettle may be a trick to harvest, it is worth it for what it gives you in a medical way. Nettle is chock-full of vitamins, minerals, and nutrients and also has a very pleasant taste that can help with a lot of your digestion and urinary health as well.

Many people worry about how the barbs will sting too much and that it isn't worth the effort to harvest fresh nettles, and you can just purchase dried nettles to save yourself the trouble; however, fresh nettles have the powerful antioxidants and other health benefits already available, and many of these vital nutrients are diminished in the drying and long term storage process. The leaves are the most important part and you do not need to concern yourself with the roots and stems at all at this point. When you harvest a nettle plant, wear protective gloves so that they are easier to handle. When you get them home, if you prefer to harvest them yourself, you can dip each leafy stalk into a stockpot of hot water to soften all of the bristles and hairs that sting. This method is known as blanching which is an oft used cooking technique for a variety of leafy greens.

Once you have gently blanched the nettles you can dry them hanging upside down, sauté and eat them fresh and cooked, or you can make an extraction.

Nettle has the following health benefits: a rich source of antioxidants, minerals, vitamins, and nutrients; provides an energetic boost to the immune system; balances digestion; aids in healthy waste elimination; stimulates the gallbladder and kidneys.

Ways to prepare Nettle: after harvesting, blanche and either eat after a gentle sauté with other ingredients, make an extraction (see Chapter 2 for instructions) or hang up to dry and then store for future use as a tea infusion. You can also make a salve with nettles and use it on irritated skin as well as on insect bites, welts, bruises, sores, cuts, and scrapes.

Parsley

Parsley is used all over the world as a garnish. In all restaurants, it is stocked in the inventory to add a little sprig to the side of the plate to make it look beautiful, but most people discard it and don't think to eat it at all. The parsley that you find in your local grocery store has usually been in cold storage for a long time, as parsley is rather hardy and can last a little longer than some other herbs can in clod storage, and so if you are able to grow it yourself at home, you will get a better benefit out of it.

Parsley is an incredibly valuable herb because of the way it cleanses your blood and your arteries. The plant is very valuable as an anticoagulant, and all you have to do is eat it every day to receive that benefit. The most healthful way to consume it is through the digestive system rather than any other way and that also includes making it into an infusion and also an extraction. Parsley can be slowly simmered over a long period of time (extraction) or lightly blanched like a tea and either will have a powerful impact on your body's health.

Parsley has the following health benefits: anticoagulant; digestive aid; blood purifier.

Ways to prepare parsley: eaten by freshly chopping and adding to the top of foods as well as cooking it with soups, stews, and sautéing it with other ingredients. Parsley tea infusion or extraction (see Chapter 2).

Rosemary

Oh, rosemary. Who on Earth hasn't heard of this magical garden herb? This plant has always worked in a lot of culinary dishes but also as a powerful healing remedy because of its potent flavor, aroma, and ability to cure a significant number of internal as well as external ailments. It is one of your go-to remedies for all issues and can sit right next to Mugwort on the shelf as regular medicine for general good health.

Rosemary grows as a thick and hardy shrub and can often be seen as a landscaping plant, but all of the landscaped gardens in the world can't undo how magical this plant actually is and how it is truly meant to be used as a medicine. The shrub-like plant has all of its power in the leaves and the thick, woody stems are rarely used for medicinal purposes. It is best to just clip stalks off the bush and harvest I small batches, leaving the bulk of the shrub intact so that you can continue to let it grow and continuously provide you with healing herb.

Rosemary has the following health benefits: ensures a proper action of the arterial cavities in the heart and the pumping of the blood; dissolves fat well in the body when eaten with your meals; protects the body against harmful bacteria and antibodies; peels away all layers of arterial heart blockages one layer at a time when consumed on a regular basis and used in correlation with a healthy diet; brings energy to the pancreatic actions and help stimulate the mucous membranes of the digestive tract; blood purifier; detoxifying agent.

Ways to prepare Rosemary: This powerful food is best enjoyed as a culinary herb and should be added to a variety of your meals and dishes. Other methods of preparing a rosemary tea or extraction become too bitter and unpleasant to taste and hard to consume at all. Eat it and enjoy its magical healing abilities!

Sage

A lot like rosemary, Sage has a lot of culinary uses and is most often seen as an herb for flavoring foods; however, sage has a long history of working its magic in other powerful ways. The sage plant has a fairly hearty plant growth with thick, woody stems and soft, fuzzy leaves that have a very earthy scent. The aroma of sage is also used as a relaxation oil, so you might be able to guess from that alone what some of its beneficial healing properties might be. The sage leaf is notable in its ability to help soothe aches and pains in the muscles, joints, and ligaments of the body and also has a way of relieving stress when consumed at a regular level of enjoyment. Like its friends Chamomile and Lavender, this plant works to help you destress, calm, soothe, relax and sleep. Not only that, Sage has a powerful level of antioxidants as well and can promote a healthy internal balance when working on a long-term health goal. Most people only see it as an occasionally useful culinary herb, but if you were to enjoy more regularly, you might find more pleasure in its relaxing abilities.

Sage has the following health benefits: helps to calm and relax the nervous system; soothes sore muscles, joints, bones, and ligaments as well as connective tissues and fascia; provides a flavorful way to promote longevity because of its antioxidant qualities; brings about a heavier sleep when taken at the end of the day.

Ways to prepare sage: Sage can be cooked with all of your favorite poultry dishes and has a great way of flavoring certain soups and stews with a savory richness and earthiness. You can also dry the leaves by Hanging and Drying and use them for making a tea infusion. Avoid using sage for extractions or essences.

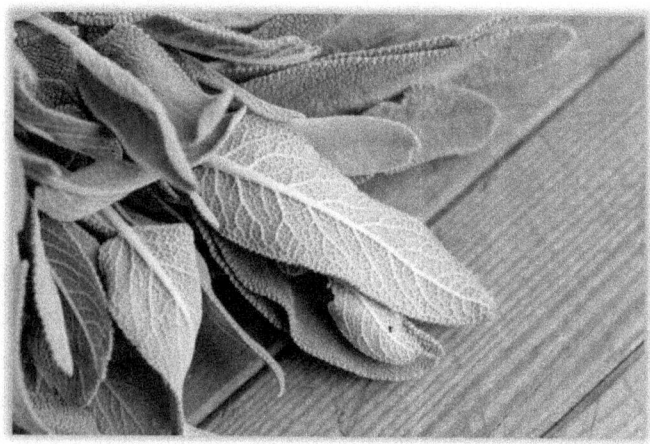

St. John's Wort

This lovely little plant has been called the best herbal anti-depressant around. St. John's Wort has a variety of uses; however, this is its main claim to fame. It has a powerful ability to restore the serotine levels of the brain's chemistry and is a remarkable way to shift mood swings into a more positive and jolly direction. Many people who practice using herbal remedies already know how awesome this little flowering plant can be and work with it often as an anti-depressant, but it has a lot of other unique qualities for a plant.

For example, St. John's Wort has also been known to help treat cancer in a number of patients, before and after receiving chemotherapy. All of the powerful minerals and antioxidants in this herb are closely linked to the health of the body on the cellular level and each little cell that has cancerous resistance to drugs will improve acceptance of cancer treatment medication with the addition of a daily, or several times daily dose of St. John's Wort. The plant itself has only leaves and some flowers at the tip, but a wonderful way to enjoy it other than making it into a tea for drinking is to simply chew on it for a little while, but never swallow it while it is fresh. It could cause nausea if consumed without drying it and steeping and infusion or extraction.

<u>St. John's Wort has the following health benefits</u>: anti-depressant; cancer-fighting abilities; antifungal; antiseptic.

Ways to prepare St. John's Wort: You can chew on it fresh but never swallow it because it can cause nausea; Dry the leaves and flowers of the plant be Hanging and Drying and concoct a tea infusion or an extraction. You can also use the flowers to create and essence.

Thyme

Thyme has a lovely earthy flavor and subtle sweetness that is often used for cooking and matches well with certain meats and vegetables. It can also be a very useful herb when making broths, soups, and stews, but it is rarely used in other ways. A lot of the benefits of this plant are thought to be only related to the flavor of food; however, it has a lot of medicinal qualities that are often overlooked, and you can almost always find it in the kitchen garden as a remedy.

Thyme can be dried and made into a tea and is a wellness tonic for a variety of medical conditions. It has an ability to alter your internal practices of how you work your lymphatic system and how your blood flows well with your lymph flow. The power of thyme is that it gives a glow to the skin and hair as well and as an additive to shampoos and conditioners, as well as facial cleansers, it can leave a rich and healthy glow to these areas.

<u>Thyme has the following health benefits</u>: Thyme is a flavoring for foods that also helps your digestion; lymphatic drainage in correlation with healthy blood flow; tonic for the skin and hair; thyme works well with all other herbs when making a concoction so be sure to add it to your herbal blend remedies as well.

<u>Ways to prepare Thyme</u>: you can dry it and use it as a cooking herb, or use it fresh for cooking. You can also use it as a dried herb to make a tea or an extraction to drink for your lymph flow or to add to your hair and skin care products.

HERBAL MEDICINE

Turmeric

An essential herb for the at-home apothecary, yet often overlooked, turmeric is packed full of quality health and healing properties. Not many people cook with it in American culture, but it has a wide variety of uses in many other cultures and is considered a staple culinary food item and is used often for both cooking and health purposes. The little roots are an orange color and when cut leaves a yellowish stain on the skin. This root was and still is used for a variety of color dyes to add the natural yellow to other items, such as colorful clothes and fabrics.

Turmeric, when cooked with, is usually seen in a powder form and is sold this way at the supermarket. You may use this form of the herb, and although it seems like a lot to use when you are making a tea for an ailment, you will need at least ¼ cup of powdered turmeric to help you with your herbal practice. The best way to use this medicine is to use the fresh roots and to make your decoctions with them this way for the best results with herbal medicine.

Turmeric has the following health benefits: anti-inflammatory for the entire system; blood purifier; overall herb for long life and vitality.

Ways to prepare Turmeric: the best way to get the most healing benefit from this magical root is to make a decoction by skinning the root and then cutting it into small pieces, bring to a boil in 1 cup of water or more depending on your needs, and then simmering

HERBAL MEDICINE

on low for 10-20 minutes. Use as many as 2-10 roots for each tonic you make and add a little lemon and 1 tsp of honey to flavor the earthy taste.

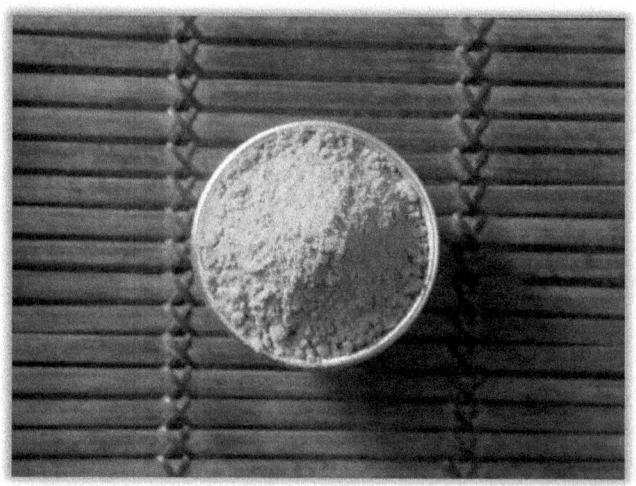

Witch Hazel

This magic herb has been widely used and widely known for centuries. It has a strange little dark-colored flower with yellow speckles and grows on the branches of a small bush like tree. The witch hazel bark is also very useful for its strong quality to cleanse and purify toxins from the skin and body.

Witch hazel is mainly used in modern times as a facial astringent or toner to help keep the skin alkaline and balanced. The external uses of witch hazel are around for today's market, and it has also been known to help heal a variety of internal issues as well. Many lifetimes ago, people who practiced witchcraft were seen as a harm to those who listened to the word of the Lord around healing and herbal remedies and so if you had knowledge about how to heal through plant magic, you were considered evil or a friend of the devil. In today's world, herbal remedies are more widely accepted than they used to be and the way witch hazel had helped so many back then was that it could clean and heal an infected wound in a very quick and easy way, much to the surprise of the lords and ladies of the time and their religious affiliates.

<u>Witch hazel has the following health benefits</u>: cleans and purifies ailments of the skin including contusions, lacerations, scars, scrapes, burns, cuts, boils, carbuncles, and warts as well as an internal healing agent to promote the ability to heal these issues from the inside working out.

<u>Ways to prepare Witch Hazel</u>: Flower Essences for internal use; decoctions made from the bark to take as tea or to apply to affected skin; flower and bark cooked down as an extraction to drink or apply to wounds; astringent made from the bark through a simmering decoction and alcohol preparation (1 oz to 1 cup of bark tea).

Yarrow

Yarrow has a big, broad flower head that looks like a soft head of a flat mushroom cap and it has a strong earthly sweet aroma. Yarrow has a variety of colors, but the one most often used as an herbal remedy is yellow yarrow. It has had a long history of use in treating loss of blood from severe wounds in the skin and was also a very popular herb during the Civil War because of its ability to staunch the flow of blood when applied directly to a wound, contusion or cut.

Yarrow works externally to slow and even stop the flow of blood, and as a contradiction to that rule of thumb, when taken internally, yarrow has a significant ability to increase the flow of blood to aid in excellent circulation. It has a way of providing for the blood in more ways than one and will always come in handy when dealing with such issues. It is also a powerful antifungal and has a bitter flavor when consumed as a tea infusion which helps with the production of healthy bile to aid in proper digestion of fats and proteins.

<u>Yarrow has the following health benefits</u>: antifungal; external blood coagulant; internal anticoagulant of the blood and promotes excellent blood flow; aids in the good bile production as a powerful bitter remedy.

<u>Ways to prepare Yarrow</u>: Always best as a tea infusion from the dried flowers only, and can also be made into an essence and an extraction.

HERBAL MEDICINE

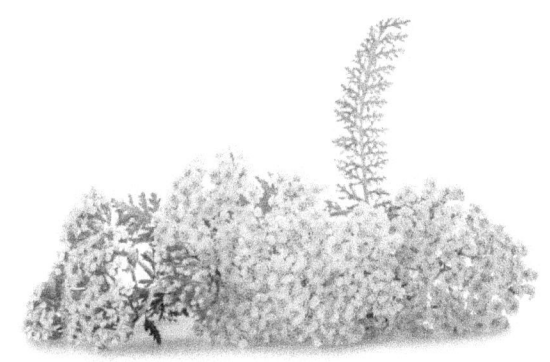

Problematic Herbs to Avoid for Safety:

Some herbs can be trickier than others when it comes to safe healing remedies. A majority of herbs are safe for consumption on a regular or semi-regular basis; however, some are a little too toxic when used in an incorrect manner. Here is a simple list of a few herbs to avoid unless you are feeling very well educated and confident about how to use in them in the proper manner:

- Belladonna
- Bittersweet
- Comfrey
- Foxglove
- Hemlock
- Ipecac
- Lily of the Valley
- Mandrake

HERBAL MEDICINE

- Mistletoe
- Pennyroyal
- Poke Root

There are several different kinds of plant species that need further study before taking them internally. All of the herbs listed in this book are safe to ingest and only one or two have a note of caution about using them in strong doses or quantities too often.

Listen to your intuition and keep an herbal field guide handy to keep you at your healthiest, safest and most knowledgeable about the plant medicine world.

CHAPTER 5

REMEDIES AND RECIPES

The next step will be to take all that you have learned from this book so far and start to apply it to make your very own, personal remedies that are just right for you and your needs. A lot of the herbs you have found in this book will be a great way to begin, however in your personal journey with healing and health you may find other herbs through your own research that are better suited to your specific needs.

Much of the lesson on health has a great deal to do with your everyday diet and so before you get started with using herbal medicine it is important to understand that you will also need to arrange to eat a diet that will support the healing benefits of herbal medicine. If you are asking yourself how to heal well in a natural way, then you are going to have to make some changes to your diet if you haven't already.

HERBAL MEDICINE

Here is a list of things to avoid in your healthy diet at all times if possible, but there are always occasions and events that are negotiable:

- Sugar- unless it comes from fruit or raw honey. Avoid artificial sweeteners as well.

- Caffeine- bye bye coffee. Sorry. It just isn't good for anyone every single day. You can treat yourself once or twice a week, but other than that, try to stick to herbal morning drinks. Also, caffeinated teas, like Earl Grey and Jasmine Tea should be avoided every day. Treat yourself to these caffeinated teas 1-2 times a week as well.

- Wheat- yes, I know. Everything has wheat in it, but all-purpose flour is a health risk and causes a lot of issues including early onset dementia and Alzheimer's, Parkinson's, certain cancers, and a slew of other illnesses and diseases that our health food industry is only just now beginning to recognize and report on.

- Alcohol- every so often, alcohol can actually be useful to your body, but it should not be consumed on a daily basis. It is the number one cause of organ system failure in our lives and many people are asking for trouble with their life-long health with this poisonous chemical.

- All Processed Foods, especially with a long list of ingredients that you have never heard of- stick to the fresh produce department, lean meats and fresh fish, eat healthy fats like olive oil, grass-fed butter, coconut oil, and avocados, even use some of these fats to flavor your healing herbs, as healthy fat help your body digest and absorb your herbal nutrients better. If you are getting things from boxes and cans, bags of chips and regularly feeding yourself from the frozen food aisle, then herbal remedies are not going to help you as a long-term health plan.

What you eat you are, and if you want to be a box of instant mashed potatoes, then you will become that pile of fluff that actually only contains a fraction of real potatoes and is also a lot of other ingredients that don't belong in your body, especially if you are trying to heal and stay well so that you can live a long and happy life.

Now that you have a clearer idea of how you need to start feeding your body overall, you can begin to open your cabinet and start to create some at home remedies and recipes that will help you with your powerful medicinals. The following list of recipes are simple ways for you to get a basic understanding of how and when to use certain herbs for certain treatments. As you become more practiced with your medicine cabinet, you can alter and modify these basic recipes to

HERBAL MEDICINE

help you create the perfect tonic, tea, extraction or essence for your humble home needs.

NOTE Be sure to use sterilized tools, containers and utensils when making and preserving these remedies. You can hot steam your containers and pots in your dishwasher, or you can pour boiling water over everything you will use. In order to keep these remedies fresh and safe for the body, you need to start with a clean workspace and tools for your project.

***(these measurements are almost always using dried herbs. For fresh herbs increase 1 TBSP to 1 cup)

Basic Cough Syrup Recipe

Ingredients:

1 lb of dried elderberries

1 Cup of dried elderberry flowers

1 lb of fresh blackberries

2 cups of raw honey

Instructions:

1. Put a pot of clean water on the stove and bring to a boil (about 2 Quarts)

2. Add elderberries and washed blackberries and turn heat down to low.

3. Simmer for an hour on low.

4. Strain berries from liquid.

5. Return liquid to the pot and add honey.

6. Melt honey and let cool.

7. Bottle and refrigerate for 2 months maximum.

8. Use during a cough 1-8 times daily in small doses (1 oz, or shot glass at a time)

Basic Throat Coat Recipe (for sore throats)

Ingredients:

1 oz dried marshmallow root (chopped into small bits)

1 oz licorice root (chopped into small bits)

3 TBSP dried sage

1 tsp honey

1 tsp lemon juice

1 garlic clove, smashed

¼ tsp fresh ginger

Instructions:

1. Add ingredients to a shallow pot or pan and add 8-16 oz of water.

2. Bring to a boil and then turn down to a simmer, stirring herbs occasionally.

3. Reduce heat as low as it goes and let sit for 15-20 minutes.

4. Strain herbs and add honey and lemon to the liquid.

5. Drink as a tea or let cool for a little while and use as a gargle.

Add warm salt water, lemon, honey, and apple cider vinegar gargle into your daily health care regimen with this tea and soothe that sore throat away.

Basic Cold and Flu Remedy

Ingredients:

10 cloves of garlic

1 lemon

1 cup of parsley, chopped

Honey to add some sweetness

16 oz of clean water

Instructions:

1. Chop the garlic coarsely and add to pot with water; bring to a boil.

2. Lower heat to a soft simmer and allow the garlic heat for 10-12 minutes.

3. Add parsley and continue simmering for another 10 minutes.

4. Strain herbs from liquid.

5. Add honey and lemon juice to garlic parsley decoction.

6. Drink several times per day during a cold or flu.

You can also add a healing broth to this health care plan, alternating between Garlic Parsley Tea and a healing, salty broth. The best way to heal during an intense cold or illness is to eat fewer large meals and consume lighter meals throughout the day. This kind of herbal remedy along with a hot cup of broth several times a day will be all you need to help you heal and keep you well nourished.

Warm and Cozy Remedy

Ingredients:

1 tsp olive oil

7 cloves of garlic, chopped

1 TBSP grated ginger

1 fresh pepper, sliced (habanero or jalapeño will work)

Zest of lemon

1 tsp of cinnamon (freshly grated is preferable)

12 oz of water

Instructions:

1. Bring water to a boil in a pot and add garlic, ginger, pepper, lemon zest and cinnamon.
2. Turn down to a simmer and let herbs heat in the water on low for 10-20 minutes.
3. Strain herbs from liquid and drink.

You can add a little honey, but don't overdo it. Too much sweet will counteract the spiciness. This is a great remedy when you are having a hard time warming up internally, or if you have an endless craving for spicy foods.

Astringent Recipe

Ingredients:

1 TBSP witch hazel bark

1 cup fresh witch hazel flowers, or ¼ cup dried

16 oz of clear, pure water (preferably not from a plastic bottle or out of your tap, distilled is best)

1 oz of high-quality alcohol (not rubbing alcohol)

Instructions:

1. Add water to a clean saucepan and add bark and flowers.

2. Let soak for 30 minutes to an hour.

3. Bring to a boil and then lower heat to a simmer for 10 minutes.

4. Strain and let cool.

5. Incorporate alcohol for preservation.

6. Use a sterilized container to store the astringent.

7. Apply to facial care program, and also use on itches, scrapes, insect bites and other skin quality concerns. Use a cotton ball to dab it on.

Basic Salve for Cuts, Burns and Bruises

Ingredients:

¼ cup beeswax chips

1 cup of olive oil

1 cup of dried arnica flowers, mugwort, or comfrey

Instructions:

1. In a pan (one you don't mind getting beeswax all over) melt your way and add your olive oil

after the wax has fully melted, keeping it at a low heat to simmer lightly.

2. Add your arnica flowers and stir them into the oil.

3. Let simmer with wax and oil for 10-15 minutes.

4. Remove from heat and strain flowers from oil.

5. Pour into a sterilized container and let cool.

6. Apply as needed to cuts, burns, and bruises on the skin.

7. You don't need to refrigerate this salve unless you want it to get harder and less soft for application purposes.

Tonic for Bowel Discomfort

Ingredients:

8 oz of barley water (see Barley in Essential Herbs Chapter 4)

1 bunch of fresh parsley

2 TBSP dried Mugwort

2 TBSP dried nettle

HERBAL MEDICINE

1 lemon, juiced

1 tsp of honey

Instructions:

1. Instead of using pure or distilled water, use the barley water to make a decoction with the parsley, nettle, and Mugwort, simmering on low for 10-15 minutes.

2. Remove from heat and strain.

3. Add honey and lemon and stir together.

4. Drink several times a day while symptoms last.

Tonic for Vitality

Ingredients:

1 TBSP angelica

1 TBSP basil

1 TBSP Mint

1 TBSP St. John's Wort

1 TBSP grated fresh ginger

1 TBSP grated fresh turmeric

1 lemon

HERBAL MEDICINE

3 cloves of garlic, smashed

Instructions:

1. Add the turmeric, garlic, and ginger to a pan of water and simmer on low after bringing to a boil for 10 minutes. Be sure to use 10-16 oz of water.

2. After the ingredients have simmered, add the lemon juice. Strain out the garlic, turmeric, and ginger.

3. Put the loose, dried herbs into a strainer (or you can also just add them directly to your teapot and strain the herbs while you pour your tea)

4. Pour the turmeric/garlic/ginger/lemon tea into the teapot (or over the dried herbs) and let steep for at least 10-15 minutes.

5. Strain herbs and serve.

6. You can let the tonic cool off to room temperature and add ice to make it a refreshing warm-weather vitality drink.

CHAPTER 6

APPLICATIONS

All herbal medicine asks is that you listen to your body and listen to the plants. What does that even mean, you may wonder? Well, all medicine has a way of communicating with you how it can help you. There is a whole world of plant-based materials that can show you exactly what they are used for when you look at their flowers, stems, roots, and branches. It's like looking at a person who has a costume on: they are clearing showing off the fact that they are a witch, or a clown, or a cowboy. Plants have a way of doing a similar thing if you pay close enough attention.

The herbs that you have read about in this book each have uniquely distinct appearances, scents, flavors and even ways of looking at you from the kitchen counter when you are feeling a certain way. Don't understand what I mean? Well, when you are craving something in your life, like garlic, ginger or parsley, your intuition and instinct have a funny way of looking directly at those items in order to alert you to the fact that you want them on a deeper level. It is how you can ascertain certain parts of your needs when you are feeling unwell, or even if you are in the prime of your health but your body is wanting a certain kind of energy or herbal concoction to help you even further or prevent getting sick in the future.

Trusting your intuition can take a little practice, but when you start paying attention to the subtle cues from your body's alerts, messages, and cravings, you can determine which herb your body is wanting most at any given moment. Let's use an example of what this might look like:

Let's say you have been doing really well with a healthy diet, have cut out caffeine, sugars, alcohol and processed foods and are feeling at the top of your health game. Meanwhile, you have been using a variety of medicinal herbs to boost your immune system, replenish your mineral and vitamin content and improve your quality of overall life and health.

Then, you ask yourself, what am I missing? Is there something my body is asking for or needing that I can give to it? What are my thoughts about when I think about food or remedies? AM I satisfied with the flavors and tastes, or the way I feel afterward?

When you ask yourself these kinds of questions, you are beginning to act on your intuition to help you discover the practice of letting your body inform you of what you need the most. This can take a lot of time and practice, but it's worth it in the long run. In this case, you may be feeling incredibly healthy but you have a regular craving for something spicy. Craving spicy foods will mean that your body is looking for heat. Rather than going out to a restaurant and ordering the spiciest dish, or pouring hot sauce from a bottle all over your rice and vegetables (which has a lot of processed foods and chemicals that will disturb your general health care plan), you can give your body the heat it is asking for through the use of herbs.

A heat tonic from Chapter 5 would be the perfect remedy to help you warm up your insides and you can improve the overall quality of your health by simply responding to that simple, subtle message with the right herbal remedy.

The most amazing thing about working with herbs is that you can offer them an understanding of how well you are when you take them and then they will show you what you need in order to continue to improve. Most of us are too busy or distracted to fully pay attention to our bodies and the herbs that are here to heal them, and that is why if you are going to teach yourself the ancient wisdom of healing with herbs you will need to begin your practice of hearing your body.

The lessons from your body are always very obvious, but to the everyday person, we are all either looking at other options to heal ourselves or completely ignoring the information our bodies are trying to communicate. As a result of too much internet research, television watching, social media scrolling, and PlayStation playing, our minds are directed significantly far away from our ability to hear the words and expressions coming from our body's feelings.

Just as you would guess that people are programmed a certain way to eat, drink, survive, and sleep, we are also programmed to evolve, and we are currently evolving in a destructive direction, avoiding the true rhythms of nature and our health. We are always in accordance with the laws of nature, no matter how much technology we incorporate into our daily lives and so it is of utmost importance that we continue to listen to how our bodies want to be treated and what will be the best way to heal them.

Medicinal herbs are always available and are usually a lot cheaper than prescription drugs and the more you acquaint yourself with the power of each little herb, flower, root, and stem, the more you will understand the best methods for attacking colds and viruses, healing your digestive system, detoxing and cleansing, preventing cancer, isolating areas of concern and treating them directly, empowering your immune system, and overall creating a very potent preventive health care plan that will ensure a long and healthy life.

While there are still so many unfortunate ideas circulating around the internet and medical circles, you can begin to apply all of the tools grown in your own backyard to enrich your whole life with health and the magic of herbal remedies. We are always going to work with the plants of this world and they will always offer the same medicine that they always have. Nothing has changed since the dawn of discovering the medical uses of herbs, and normally, people would have all of this knowledge still readily available to them like brushing your teeth or tying your shoes. Until we are ready to remember that these are the first medicines and they will always be the most helpful to us, we are going to be faced with a lot of internal disturbances and health problems.

Applying an herbal remedy to all of your health and eating experiences will ensure you with the longevity you are looking for. Try a new diet to help you lose or gain weight, with all of that going on in your body and then add a lot of herbs that support weight loss or gain, help detox the body, stretch your intestinal lining to help you release trapped toxins and purge wastes that cause you to perform at lower levels of body strength. Any health practice can be complemented by the use of herbs. Diet and exercise are such a huge part of our cultural beliefs and reality about how to live well and healthfully, but unless you are adding healing herbs to your diet on a regular basis to boost all of your internal performance systems, you may not be acting as healthfully as you think.

To compliment any diet and exercise routine with the right herbs, all you need to do is know the herbs and what they will offer to you. Knowing that arnica rubs will help with muscle soreness, after a heavy lifting workout at the gym, you can bring your homemade salve to the locker room and apply it to your muscle

HERBAL MEDICINE

groups you know will be sore in the morning as a preventive care measure. You can reapply when there is soreness and before returning to your exercise plan.

Other applications for these herbal remedies exist in every moment of the day. When you wake up groggy and feel like you didn't get enough sleep, don't drink coffee, make a Tonic of Vitality to get your blood flowing (see Chapter 5). If you are feeling restless at night and are having a hard time winding down, make an herbal tea blend of Lavender, Sage, Basil, and Chamomile to help your whole system flow into a more relaxed state so that you can drift off to sleepy town.

You don't have to be an expert to use these herbs, and once you begin to practice with them more, you will get a better understanding of how they can affect and impact your life. When you go to your local tea or herbal remedy store, ask the people who work there if they have recommendations for certain ailments or issues. You can learn a large amount from the people in your local community who are also practicing with the herbs and learning about how they will best serve you.

Each time you go to the shop or look online, try something new and see how it feels. The best way to understand these herbs is to let them show you their qualities, properties, and characteristics by taking them in one at a time and truly exploring the benefits. You may find that one week of making a Turmeric decoction helps relieve your arthritis and that you no longer are in need of your prescription drug to relieve that discomfort. It all has to happen at a slow pace over time so that your body can rebalance to help you stay in equilibrium.

Many people practice herbal medicine without a sense of patience, and this can be the reason people give up their studies. These remedies are not instant fixes, and they require some devotion, time, space and love. When you are ill, you can quickly soothe yourself with a hot cup of broth and a Basic Cold and Flu Remedy Tea, but you have to continue to apply these herbs to your body every day at least 2-3 times in order to receive the full benefit of their powerful healing properties.

What you gain in health is worth the time and energy it takes to look at all of these herbs and what they can do to support you, not only right now or with this cold season, but over the course of your whole life.

HERBAL MEDICINE

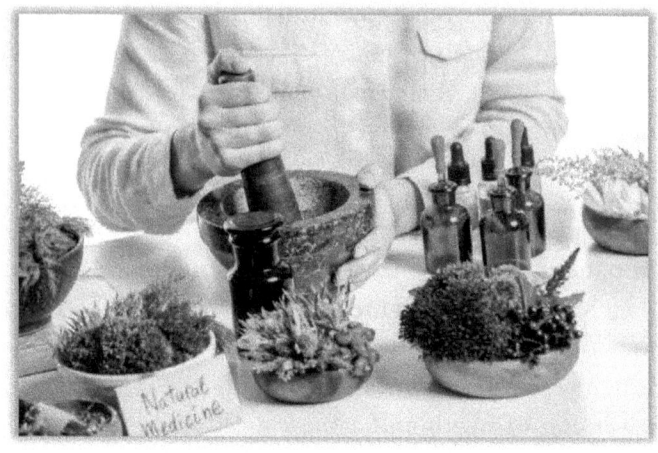

CONCLUSION

Remedies from the plant kingdom will never go out of fashion. They are here to stay and looking back at how the world has changed to embrace a culture of prescriptions and pharmaceuticals you will notice a significant increase in health issues and diseases all over civilized cultures.

The medicine cabinet in your home is promoting a life of longevity, wellness, vitality, health, productivity, love, and patience. All you need to do to help yourself live a long and healthy life is to show yourself the practice of knowing, understanding and making herbal remedies. They go hand in hand with a balanced diet, exercise, good rest and plenty of love and play.

As you go forth through your journey of healing herbs and discover more of their qualities, remember that this ancient wisdom has been around for a significant portion of our evolution as humans. It has always been a part of culture and civilization and remains to this day the best method for healing and caring for your whole-body system.

Practice getting to know each herb and acquaint yourself with others that were not mentioned in these chapters. A well-illustrated or photographed herbal field guide will come in great handy to help you learn all you need to know about the healing world of plants, flowers, roots, and leaves.

HERBAL MEDICINE

Be prepared to have fun and make a mess in your kitchen. Get creative and use some of these basic recipes to expand upon and invent your own. It is really simple to get a great idea of how you want to work with herbs and build on what you have already learned here in this book to start inventing your own personal herbal remedies that are perfectly suited to your specific needs.

All you need are some herbs, water, heat and a pot to get started. Let yourself find your favorite medicinal herbs and practice with those to start as you jump off into the wise old world of healing herbal remedies.

Finally, if you enjoyed this book and found it helpful for your needs, a honest review is always appreciated. Thank You!

www.ingramcontent.com/pod-product-compliance
Lightning Source LLC
Chambersburg PA
CBHW071719020426
42333CB00017B/2324